SET FREE

A Caregivers

Daily Devotional Journal

BEING SET FREE IS A PROCESS
LIKE A BUTTERFLY'S DEVELOPMENT

1. *Larva* — The immature form that is unlike the adult and must undergo metamorphosis.

   Metamorphosis: The complete transformation of character, purpose, and circumstances.

2. *Pupa* — The quiescent stage in the development.

   Quiescent: Being in a state of inaction.

3. *Butterfly* — Emerges in all of its God-created beauty and splendor to try its new wings - looks back - then flies free into its new life.

Cover illustration from an original watercolor by Dan Crusie, 1988.
McClain High School Art Teacher, Greenfield, Ohio ©

SET FREE

A Caregivers

Daily Devotional Journal

Martha C. Wood

LILY PUBLICATIONS

Kansas City, Missouri

Words typed in **bold face** are the compiler's emphasis.

Words typed in *italic* are the words of Jesus in the Bible.

Published by Lily Publications for
Personal Word Ministries, Inc.
11309 E. 78th Terrace
Raytown, Mo 64138

ISBN 0-9651906-3-3 $18.00

Printed in the United States of America

Then those who feared the LORD
spoke to one another,
and the LORD gave attention
and heard it,
and a book of remembrance
was written before Him
for those who fear the LORD
and who esteem His name.

Malachi 3:16 NAS

INTRODUCTION

Easter, 1981: I was recovering from surgery. I decided to use the recovery time to study Jesus' healings. I poured over Matthew, Mark, Luke, and John, writing down the who, what, where, when, why, how for each healing. I found approximately forty healing stories and a new awareness of the many different ways Christ healed.

This project was filed away until ten years later when I found myself in a personal crisis. My husband, Ron, was experiencing inexplicable behavioral changes. He was 53 years old - a high school athletic director. He was 6 feet 4 inches tall and weighed 220 lbs. He had always been in excellent health. Now Ron was diagnosed with Alzheimer's disease. Out of my strong faith, I really was in denial that anything was medically wrong with him. It was a full year before I was able to absorb the reality of Ron's disease, and it took even longer to understand its implications. It was time to review Jesus' healings and look for new insight.

This journal is born out of that quest. It is my hope that the God-given hope, courage, strength, counsel, direction, peace, and joy I received are here also for you in these pages. This journal also represents my way of working out my grief.

Aspects of the journal I think you'll enjoy include:

Biblical foundation: During Lent of 1987, a group of people at First United Methodist Church in Greenfield, Ohio, participated in "The Great Experiment." We committed to the discipline of a 5:30 A.M. daily quiet and devotional time. A life-changing process began for me as I discovered new insights into God's Word through my own scriptural reading and through various books. Each day in Scripture resulted in greater emotional and spiritual freedom.

Journaling: I discovered the joy of journaling. To share this discovery with you, I have left several spaces where you can express your own feelings. Pick up a red pen and underline, make notes, draw pictures, or communicate with God in any form that flows out of you. Many scripture passages and prayers contain blank lines. This is where you will write in your own name or the name of someone you are praying for.

Timeliness: It continually amazes me that God can speak to me through predated devotional material and study guides. I want to share that awesome feeling with you as you walk your path using these daily devotions for a year.

Illustrations: I am very childlike and simple-minded. God speaks to me in elementary pictures. They stay with me and constantly encourage me when I glance at them. May these pictures speak comfort, hope, and encouragement to you in the busy demands of your daily caregiving responsibilities.

Spiral binding: The spiral binder enables you to leave a page open each day and to meditate on the message as you pass by. I encourage you to keep this devotional in a place where you spend a lot of time during your day.

May the Word of God be sweet as honey to you. Ezekiel 3:3

Martha

JANUARY 1

When you first realize that you will be the Caregiver of a loved one, you are flooded with emotions of:

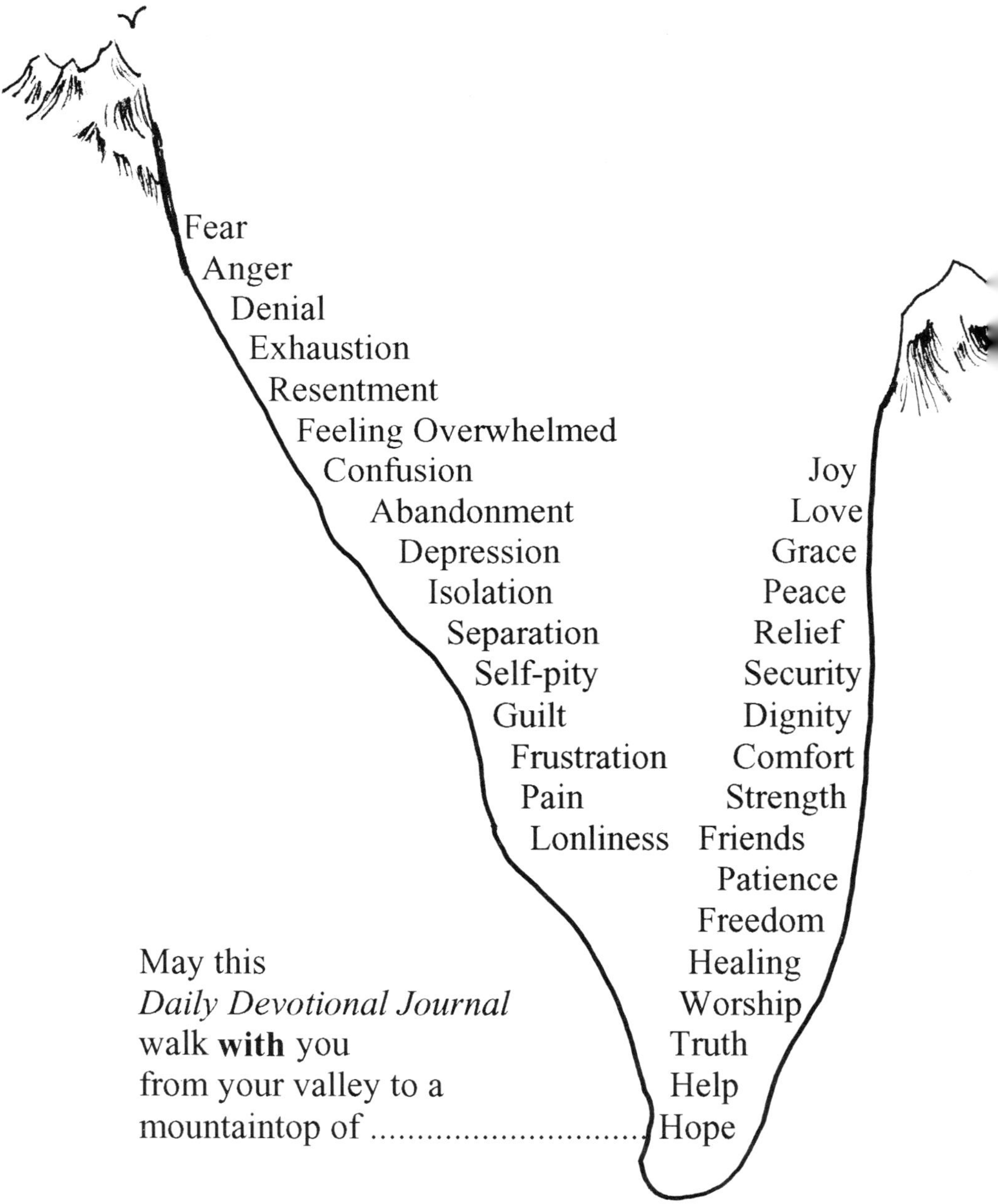

May this
Daily Devotional Journal
walk **with** you
from your valley to a
mountaintop of .... Hope

JANUARY 2

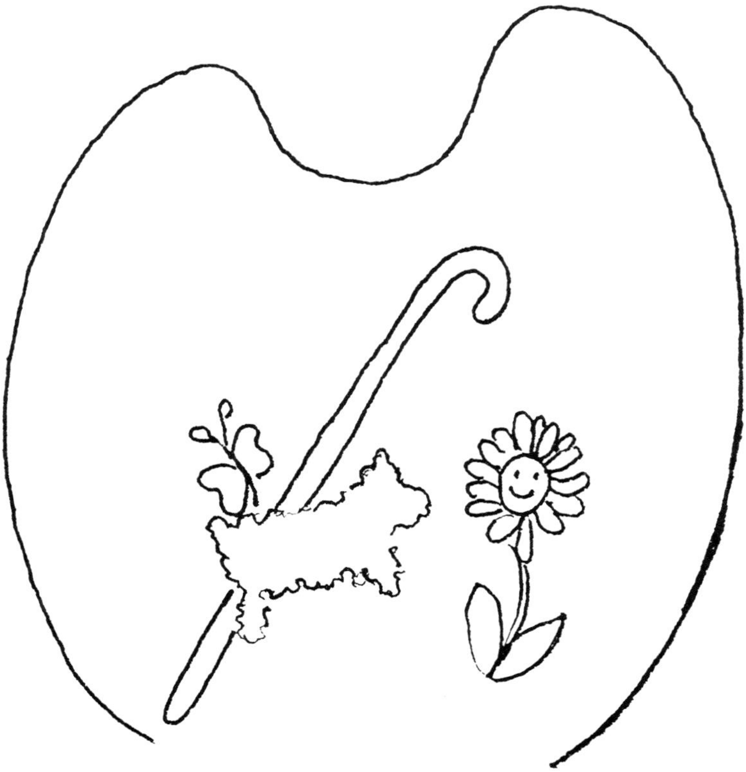

You are God's special lamb
His staff is guiding you
You will develop like a caterpillar into a butterfly
As you learn acceptance with joy
Know that God's huge arms surround you eternally

H old	**H** old
U in	**U** in
G od's Arms	**G** od's Arms
E ternally	

JANUARY 3

DISCIPLINE TO DAILY DEVOTIONAL LIFE

1. EARLY IN THE MORNING WILL I SEEK HIM

And IF My people who are called by My name
_____________themselves
____
_____________My face . . . ,
THEN I WILL
_____________from heaven,
_____________their sin,
_____________their land.

2 Chronicles 7:14 NAS

2. PLACE A LIGHTED CANDLE BEFORE YOU

Jesus said,
"I am the light of the world;
he who ____________Me
shall not walk in the ____________,
but shall have the light of ___________."

John 8:12 NAS

3. DRINK A GLASS OF WATER

Jesus said,
". . . whoever drinks of the water
that I shall ____________him
shall ___________ ______________;
but the water that I shall give him
shall become in him a _________of __________
_____________up to eternal life.

John 4:14 NAS

JANUARY 4

4. SING PRAISE AND WORSHIP SONGS ALL DAY LONG

Let the word of Christ richly dwell __________ you,
with all wisdom____________ and ________________
one another with ___________ and ________________
and _________________ , singing with thankfulness
in your hearts to God.

Colossians 3:16 NAS

5. READ SCRIPTURE AND FROM DEVOTIONAL BOOK

I have __________ Your word in my__________
that I might not _________ against You.
O p e n my eyes that I may see
_________________things in Your___________.
Oh, how I love Your law!
I ____________ on it all ____________ long.
Your word is a ___________ to my __________
and a ____________ for my ______________.

Psalm 119:11, 18, 97, 105 NIV

6. JOURNAL DAILY Wrap your prayer requests in the circle of God's love

Praise .... Adoration of God
Confession .... Of your sins
Thanks .... For answers to prayer
Requests for .... Family, friends, others, government, worldwide concerns.

Pray around your town for churches, schools, hospitals, for people in helping organizations and occupations, government, for God to heal the cities.

JANUARY 5

Jesus traveled all through Galilee teaching in the Jewish synagogues, everywhere preaching the Good News about the Kingdom of Heaven.

And He **healed every** kind of sickness and disease.

The report of His miracles spread far beyond the borders of Galilee so that sick folk were soon coming to be healed from as far away as Syria.

And whatever their illness and pain,
or if they were possessed by demons,
or were insane, or paralyzed -

He healed them all.

Enormous crowds followed Him wherever He went -

people from Galilee, and the Ten Cities, and Jerusalem,
and from all over Judea, and even from across the
Jordan River.

Matthew 4:23-25 (TLB). See also Mark 3:7-10 and Luke 6:17-19.

JANUARY 6

LORD'S PRAYER

Our Father, who art in heaven, Hallowed be Thy name.	Go to God in reverence
Thy kingdom come.	God's control
Thy will be done, on earth as it is in heaven.	Be in His will
Give us this day our daily bread.	Ask for what you need
And forgive us our debts, as we also have forgiven our debtors.	Forgive, if you want forgiven
And do not lead us not into temptation, But deliver us from evil.	Choose the right road

For Thine is the **KINGDOM, and the POWER, and the GLORY, FOREVER!! Amen!** Matthew 6:9-13 NAS

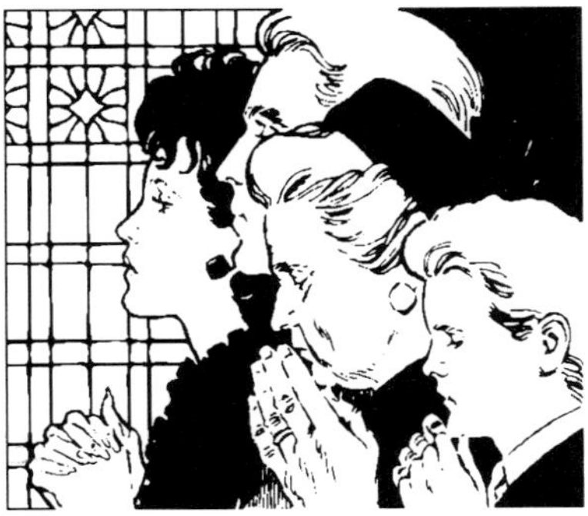

JANUARY 7

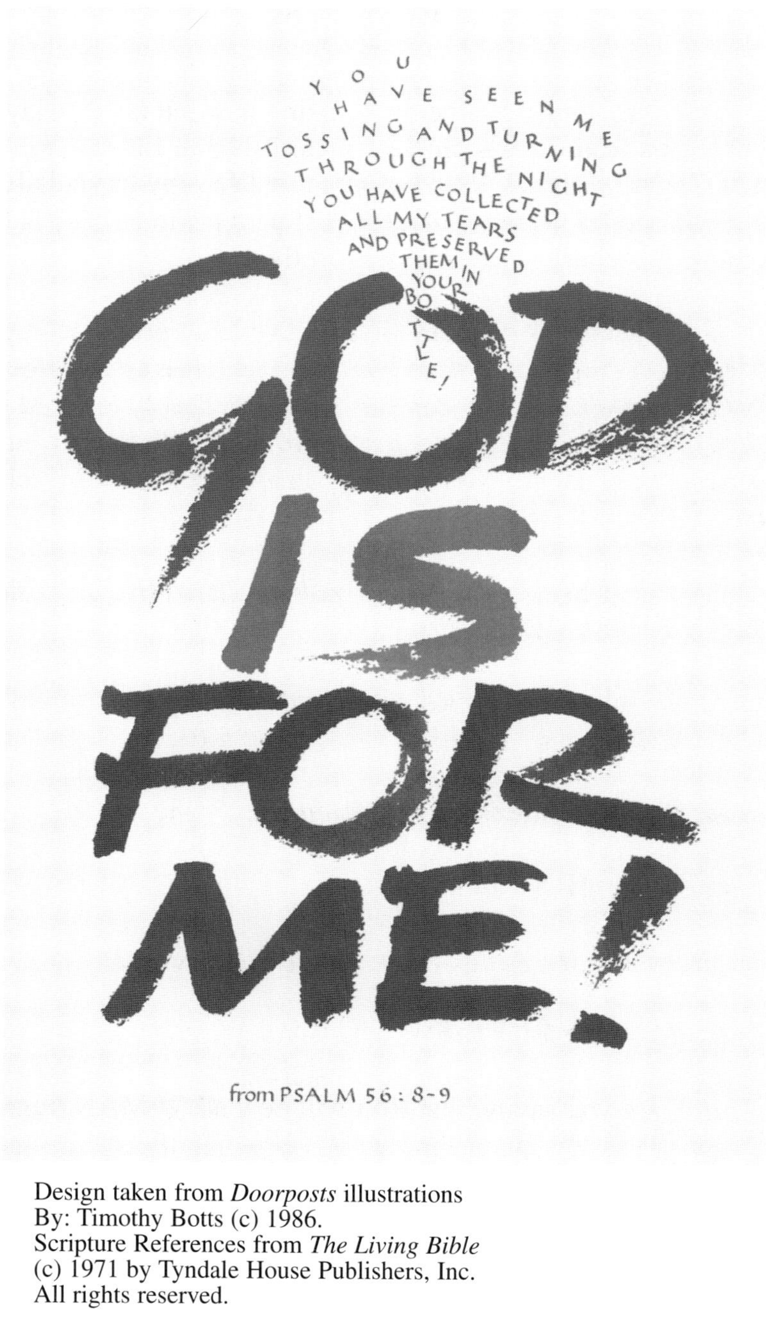

Design taken from *Doorposts* illustrations
By: Timothy Botts (c) 1986.

JANUARY 8

N E W M A N

All week long I had been preparing to teach the Sunday School lesson from John 6 on "Jesus, the Bread of Life." The truth of Christ being the Bread of my own life - my basic daily food - was beginning to sink into my being. I planned to bake bread early Sunday morning and share it with the class.

Friday was my birthday, and the Lord had prepared a special gift for me. A neighbor, whom I seldom see, came to the door with freshly baked rolls as a birthday gift. I was so deeply touched by her thoughtfulness. And I was even more excited that she would bring fresh rolls just as I was working on a "bread" Sunday School lesson.

My daughter-in-love called. After I shared this story she asked, "What is the lady's name?"

"What difference does it make? You wouldn't know her. You're in Kansas City and I am in Ohio!" I smartly retorted.

"Because God gives blessings through names," she replied.

"Oh, well, it was Helen Newman."

Silence overcame me as that name settled into my soul.

"NEWMAN . . . NEW MAN! NEW MAN!!"

"Oh, Lord, are you saying that Ron will be a NEW MAN through the Bread of Life?" In addition to the joy of that thought, what excitement I felt when I realized that God was using such a unique way of speaking to me!

JANUARY 9

JESUS TOUCHED THE UNTOUCHABLE

Large crowds followed Jesus as He came down the hillside.

Look! A leper is approaching.
He kneels before Him (Jesus)

worshiping

"Sir," the leper pleads,

"if you want to, You can heal me."

Jesus **touches** the man.

"I want to," He says. ***"Be healed."***

And **instantly** the leprosy disappears.

Then Jesus says to him,

"Don't stop to talk to anyone;
go right over to the priest to be examined;
and take with you the offering required by Moses' law
for lepers who are healed -
a public testimony of your cure."

Matthew 8:1-4 (TLB). See also Mark 1:39-45, Luke 5:12-14.

JANUARY 10

CAREGIVING JESUS IN YOUR PATIENT

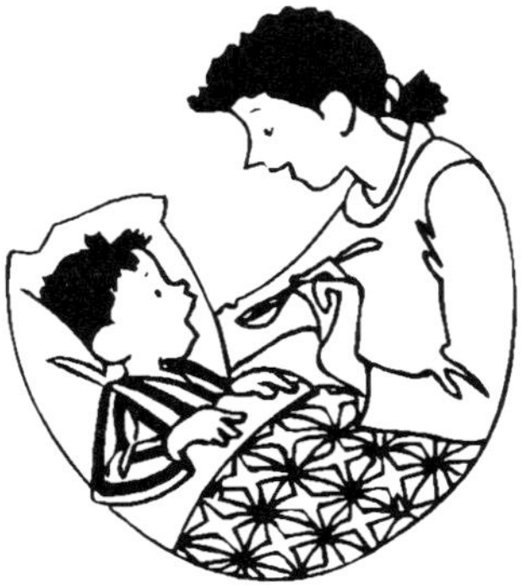

And so, as those who have been chosen of God, holy and beloved,
put on
a heart of compassion, kindness, humility,
gentleness and patience; bearing with one another,
and forgiving each other,
whoever has a complaint against anyone;
just as the Lord forgave you, so also should you.
And beyond all these things
put on love,
which is the perfect bond of unity.
And let the peace of Christ rule in your hearts . . .

Let the word of Christ richly dwell within you,
with all wisdom teaching and admonishing one another
with psalms and hymns and spiritual songs,
singing with thankfulness in your hearts to God.

And whatever you do in word or deed, do all in the name of the Lord Jesus, giving thanks through Him to God the Father.

Colossians 3:12-17 NAS

JANUARY 11

Then the Lord appeared to Solomon at night and said to him,

"I have heard your prayer,
and have chosen this place for Myself
as a house of sacrifice.

If I shut up the heavens so that there is no rain, or
if I command the locust to devour the land, or
if I send pestilence among My people,

and My people who are called by My name

humble themselves and
pray, and
seek My face and
turn from their wicked ways,

then I will

hear from heaven, will
forgive their sin, and will
heal their land.

Now My eyes shall be open and
My ears attentive to the prayer offered in this place.

For now I have chosen and consecrated this house
that My name may be there forever,
and My eyes and My heart will be there perpetually."

2 Chronicles 7:12-16 NAS

JANUARY 12

My given name is Martha Ann and today is my birthday. After my high school graduation, I longed to forget my lonely adolescence and step out anew. I began using the name *Martie.* Now I can see that it was a subconscious way to be a new person.

When I discovered who Martha was in the Bible, I knew that I lived up to my given name. I was a Martha. I was distracted with all of my preparations and had neglected to sit at Jesus' feet. I was a "Do-For" people-person. I needed to learn to become a "Be-With" people-person.

Then I discovered Anna in the Bible. I too was becoming advanced in years - I yearned to serve the Lord night and day, be in prayer, thanksgiving, and speak of Him to all who were looking for redemption.

In a baby name book I discovered that Martha means "Keeper of the House" and Ann means "Grace." I now know that both names fit my adult life roles and especially my Caregiver role. I discovered that God is faithful with blessings, even in giving us our names.

What is your name? What does it mean?

____

What is your patient's name? What does it mean?

____

You can speak a blessing over your patient by saying his or her name.

Luke 10:38-42 tells a story about Martha.
Luke 2:36-38 tells Anna's story.

JANUARY 13

HEALING OF MEMORIES PRAYER

Dear Jesus,

I ask You to enter _________ who has need of Your healing.

I rejoice that as the light of Your love now fills this mansion of_________, all darkness shall flee.

Look and see, O Lord, whether there be any ugly pictures on the walls - pictures of old distressful and horrifying wounds of the past.

And if there be such pictures, take them down and give to _________memory house - pictures of beauty and joy.

Go back, Lord, through all the rooms of this memory house.

Open every closed door and see if there be any dirty and broken thing that is no longer needed . . .

And if so, O Lord, take it away completely.

Go back even to the years of childhood . . .

Open windows long sealed and let in the gentle sunlight of Your love.

Take a broom of mercy and sweep away the shame of ancient memories as You promised in Isaiah 54:4.

Follow the soul of this Your child all the way back to the hour of birth and heal even the pain and fear of being born.

I pray that You will restore _________ soul as You made it and will quicken it in all those creative impulses that You have placed therein, so that Your purpose may be fulfilled.

I give thanks, O Lord, knowing that this healing of _________ is Your will and is the very purpose for giving of Your life for us.

And that, therefore, it is even now being accomplished.

Author unknown

JANUARY 14

. . . **Do not fear**, for those who are with us

are more than those who are with them.

2 Kings 6:16 NAS

Lord, today I am feeling like this . . .

JANUARY 15

When Jesus arrived in Capernaum, a Roman army captain came and pled with Him to come to his home and heal his servant boy who was in bed paralyzed and racked with pain.

"Yes," Jesus said, *"I will come and heal him."*

Then the officer said,

> "Sir, I am not worthy to have You in my home;
> (and it isn't necessary for You to come).
> If You will only stand here and say,
> **'Be healed,'**
> my servant will get well!
> I know, because I am under the authority of my superior officers and I have authority over my soldiers, and I say to one, 'Go,' and he goes, and to another, 'Come,' and he comes, and to my slave boy, 'Do this or that,' and he does it. And I know You have authority to tell his sickness to go - and it will go!"

Jesus stood there amazed! Turning to the crowd He said,

> *"I haven't seen faith like this in all the land of Israel! And I tell you this, that many Gentiles (Like this Roman officer), shall come from all over the world and sit down in the Kingdom of Heaven with Abraham, Isaac, and Jacob. And many an Israelite - those for whom the Kingdom was prepared - shall be cast into outer darkness, into the place of weeping and torment."*

Then Jesus said to the Roman officer,

> *"Go on home. What you have believed has happened!"*
>
> And the boy **was healed that same hour**!
>
> Matthew 8:5-13 (TLB). See also Luke 7:2-10 and John 4:46-54.

JANUARY 16

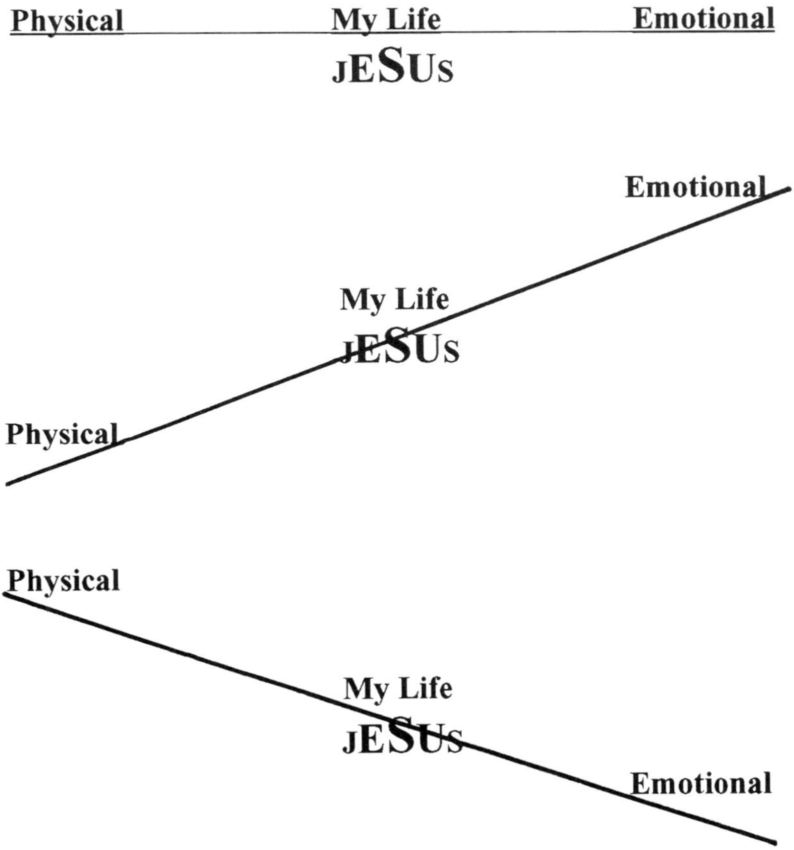

Lord, help me keep my life in **balance.**

A just balance and scales belong to the LORD;
All the weights of the bag are His concern.
Proverbs 16:11 NAS

JANUARY 17

WHY? WHY? WHY?

This is the great lesson of the book of Job in the Bible:

"If we know God, we do not need to know **why** He allows us to experience what we do. He is not only in control of the universe and all its facets but also of our lives; and **He loves us**. Though His ways are sometimes beyond our comprehension, we should not criticize Him for His dealings with us or with others.

God is always in control of all things,
even when He appears not to be."[1]

Then Job replied to God:
"I know that You can do anything and that no one can stop You.
You ask who it is who has so foolishly denied Your providence.
It is I. I was talking about things I knew nothing about
and did not understand, things far too wonderful for me.

You said,
'Listen and I will speak!
Let Me put the questions to you!
See if you can answer them!'

But now I say,
'I had **heard about You before,** but **now I have seen You,**
and I loathe myself and repent in dust and ashes.' " . . .

Then, when Job prayed for his friends,
the LORD restored his wealth and happiness!
In fact, the LORD gave him twice as much as before!

Job 42:1-6, 10 TLB

[1] Taken from: *The Ryrie Study Bible NAS* by Charles C. Ryrie, Copyright 1976, 1978, Moody Bible Institute of Chicago. Moody Press. p. 796. Used by permission.

JANUARY 18

HUGGING

HUGGING IS HEALTHY:

It helps the body's immunity system,
It keeps you healthier,
It cures depression,
It reduces stress,
It induces sleep,
It is invigorating,
It is rejuvenating,
It has no unpleasant side effects,
It is nothing less than a miracle drug.

HUGGING IS ALL NATURAL:

It is organic, naturally sweet, no pesticides,
no preservatives, no artificial ingredients,
and is 100 percent wholesome

HUGGING IS PRACTICALLY PERFECT:

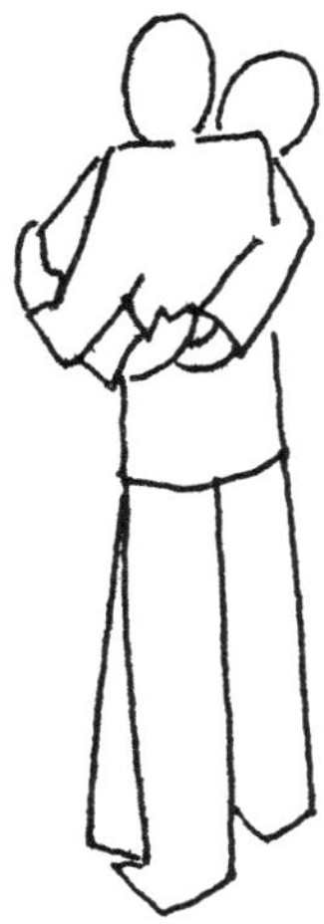

There are no movable parts,
no batteries to wear out,
no periodic checkups,
low-energy consumption,
high-energy yield, inflation-proof,
non-fattening, no monthly payments,
no insurance requirements, theft proof,
non-taxable, non-polluting and of course,
fully returnable.

Author Unknown

JANUARY 19

If you are wise,
live a life of steady goodness,
so that only good deeds will pour forth.
And if you don't brag about them,
Then **you will be truly wise!**

And by all means don't brag about being wise and good
if you are bitter and jealous and selfish;
that is the worst sort of lie.
For jealousy and selfishness are not God's kind of wisdom.
Such things are earthly, unspiritual, inspired by the devil.
For wherever there is jealousy or selfish ambition,
there will be disorder and every other kind of evil.

But the **wisdom** that comes from heaven is first of all

pure and full of quiet gentleness
then . . .
peace-loving and courteous
allows discussion
is willing to yield to others
is full of mercy and good deeds
wholehearted and straightforward
sincere

And those who are peacemakers will plant seeds of peace
and reap a harvest of goodness.

James 3:13-18 (TLB)

JANUARY 20

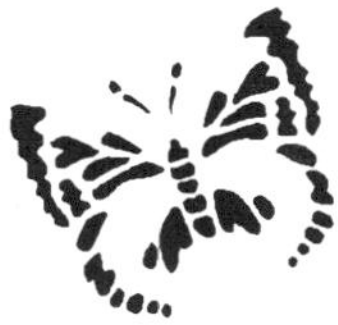

Butterflies are free

To Be

Who God wants them

To Be.

They fly with grace

and beauty,

From the old

to the new.

You will go from

High school to
college or job

Teenager to woman.

Soar gracefully

To be free
To become

GOD'S WOMAN

Fifty and free

To Be

Who God created

You to be.

Filled with years of

Love and Wisdom,

Set free to soar

to new heights

and creative ways

To share God's

Love and Wisdom.

JANUARY 21

"For I will **restore** you to health

And I will **heal** you of your wounds,"

declares the Lord . . .

Jeremiah 30:17 NAS

Lord, today I am feeling like this . . .

JANUARY 22

HEALED TO SERVE

When Jesus arrived at Peter's house,
Peter's mother-in-law was in bed with a high fever.

But when Jesus **touched** her hand,
the fever left her;
and she got up and
prepared a meal for them!

Matthew 8:14-15 (TLB). See also Mark 1:29-31 and Luke 4:38-39.

~~~~~~~~~~~~~~~~~~~~

My Pastor, Bob Campbell, made this comment about the passage:

"Makes me think of a hospital waiting room.
As people stream in and out, the volunteer asks,

'And **who** are you here for?'

Maybe that's a more important question than,

'**What** am I here for?'

Or maybe it answers it.

Who am I here for?
Who can I touch with Jesus' healing love today?"
~~~~~~~~~~~~~~~~~~~~

JANUARY 23

FOUR-LETTER WORDS

LOVE	CARE	COME	LIFE
HOME	HOPE	WELL	GROW
FOOD	FEEL	HUGS	TALK
GOOD	PRAY	KISS	SING
LIVE	HELP	GIFT	ABLE
WAIT	BABE	BATH	BOLD
BORN	CALL	CALM	DEAR
WALK	ZEAL	DRAW	WORK
WITH	FEEL	TIME	HEAL

This is a trustworthy statement;
and concerning these things
I want you to speak confidently,
so that those who have believed God

may be careful to engage in good deeds.

These things are good and profitable for men.

Titus 3:8 NAS

JANUARY 24

Yet those who **wait** for the LORD
Will gain **new strength**;

They will mount up with wings like eagles,
They will run and not get tired,
They will walk and not become weary.

Isaiah 40:31 NAS

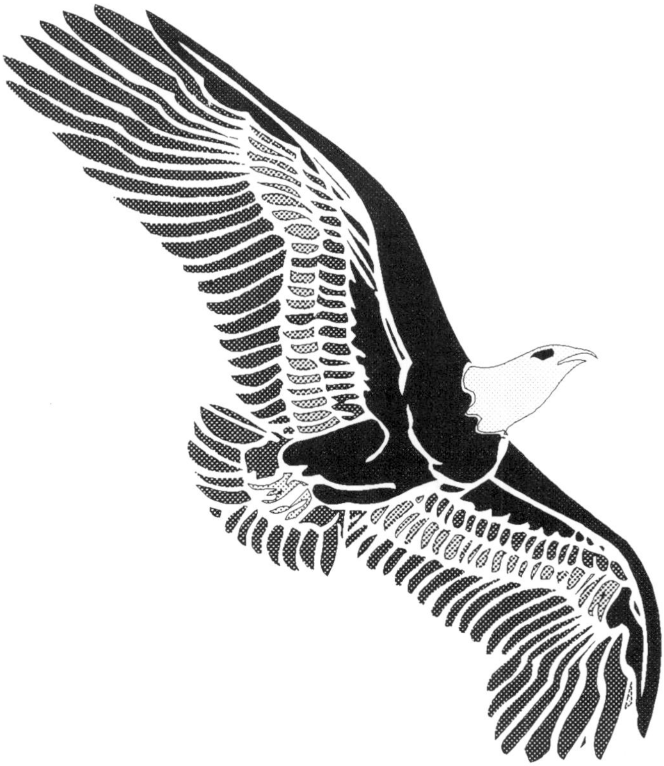

JANUARY 25

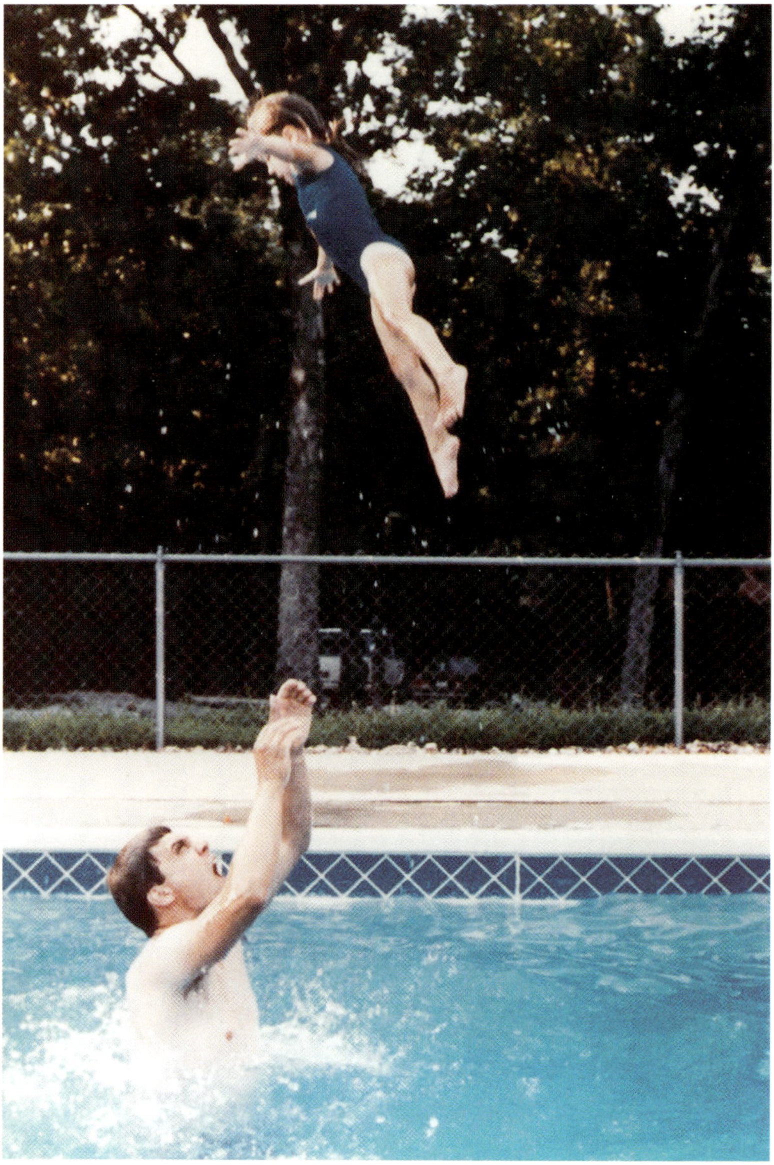

Photograph by Shannon Wood

JANUARY 26

On January 26, 1990, I received pictures in the mail that Shannon, Ron's niece, had taken while we were on vacation the previous summer.

This one picture of my son and his daughter spoke to me so clearly of my Heavenly Father's love and care for us.

See how high Rebecca is in the air? See her relaxed body? She **knows** her Dad will catch her. She completely trusts him. See the outstretched arms of Steve? He is ready to receive his daughter in joy. He may splash her, but his arms will hold her in security.

The picture spoke to me of the everlasting arms of my Heavenly Father. I **knew** I had to relax and trust the Father, even if I get splashed - The Heavenly Father will not let me drown.

The eternal God is a dwelling place,
And underneath are the everlasting arms;
And He drove out the enemy from before you,
And said, **"Destroy!"**

Deuteronomy 33:27 NAS

God, Heavenly Father, be to me The Everlasting Arms.

JANUARY 27

If therefore there is any encouragement in Christ,

if there is any consolation of love,

if there is any fellowship of the Spirit,

if any affection and compassion,

make my joy complete

by being of the same mind,

maintaining the same love,

united in spirit,

intent on one purpose.

Do nothing from selfishness or empty conceit,

but with humility of mind

let each of you regard one another as more important than himself;

do not merely look out for your own personal interests,

but also for the interests of others.

Philippians 2:1-4 NAS

JANUARY 28

But you,

be strong and do not lose courage,

for there is reward for your work.

2 Chronicles 15:7 NAS

Lord, today I am feeling like this . . .

When you run into a problem,
and you can't fight it, or flee from it,
go with the flow.

JANUARY 29

That evening several demon-possessed people
were brought to Jesus;

and when He **spoke** a single word,

all the demons fled;

and **all** the sick were **healed**.

This fulfilled the prophecy of Isaiah,

"He took our sicknesses and bore our diseases."

Matthew 8:16-17 (TLB). See also Mark 1:32-34, Isaiah 53:4-6.

JANUARY 30

J	O	Y
E	T	O
S	H	U
U	E	
S	R	
	S	

". . . What commandment is the foremost of all?"
Jesus answered, *"The foremost is, 'Hear, O Israel! The LORD our God is one LORD; and you shall* ***love the LORD your God*** *with all your heart, and with all your soul, and with all your mind, and with all your strength.' The second is this, 'You shall* ***love your neighbor*** *as yourself.' There is no other commandment greater than these."*

Mark 12:28-31 NAS

Jesus said, *"But seek first His kingdom and His righteousness; and all these things shall be added to you. Therefore do not be anxious for tomorrow; for tomorrow will care for itself."*

Matthew 6:33,34 NAS

JANUARY 31

Do not fear, for I have redeemed you;

I have called you by name; you are Mine!

When you pass **through** the **waters,**
I will be with you;

And **through** the **rivers,**
they will not overflow you.

When you walk **through** the **fire,**
you will not be scorched,
nor will the flame burn you.

For I am the LORD your God,
The Holy One of Israel, your Savior . . .

Since you are precious in My sight,
Since you are honored and I love you . . .

Do not fear, for I am **with** you.

Isaiah 43:1-5 NAS

FEBRUARY 1

COME HOLY SPIRIT COME

Come to me first as a Woman
Come to me in my role of a Wife
Come to me as I Mother my children
Come as I learn the wisdom of being a Grandmother
Come to me in the quiet of living alone.

Come Holy Spirit Come, as I strive to do Your will,
by serving in this phase of Your work of my local church.
As I now pray for the area of work that I know best,
bless my labors that they may be in Your will.

Father, it is very difficult to do Your will,
especially with those close to me who I find hard to like.
I pray now for my neighbor or family member
who really rubs me wrong.
Help me to see this person as Your child.

My deepest need right now, Father,
is to have You become the very most important One in my life.
Open my heart that I may receive Your love.

Come HOLY SPIRIT Come.

Come and pour Your healing oil of love into me
and into those I pray for.

Prayer written for a women's meeting in fall, 1972.
I would now add prayer for God's wisdom in my Caregiving role
and for healing of my loved one.

FEBRUARY 2

Jesus said,

"Therefore everyone who hears these words of Mine,
and acts upon them,
may be compared to a wise man,
who built his house upon the rock.

And the rain descended,
and the floods came,
and the winds blew,
and burst against that house;
and yet it did not fall,
for it had been founded upon the rock.

And everyone who hears these words of Mine,
and does not act upon them,
will be like a foolish man,
who built his house upon the sand.

And the rain descended,
and the floods came,
and the winds blew,
and burst against that house;
and it fell,
and great was its fall."

Matthew 7:24-27 NAS

FEBRUARY 3

HEALING COMES FROM THE INSIDE OUT

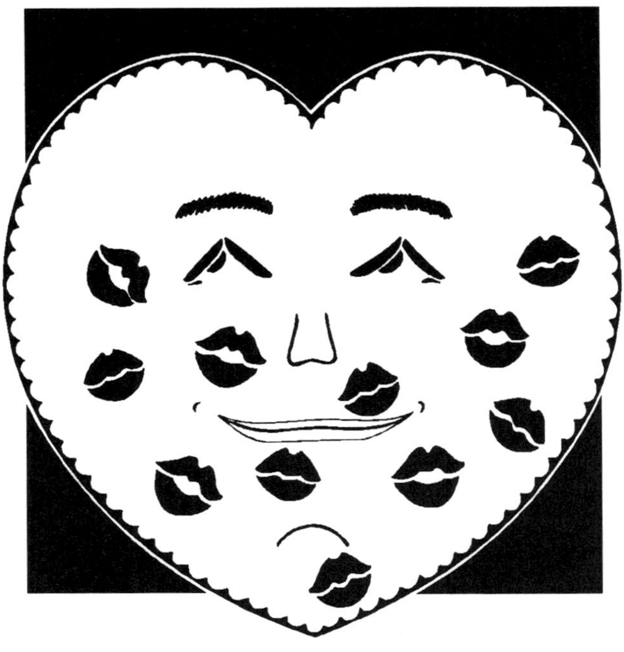

FEBRUARY 4

I went down into the orchard of nuts and
out to the **valley** to see the springtime there,
to see whether the grape vines were budding
or the pomegranates were blossoming yet.

Before I realized it I was stricken with terrible homesickness
and wanted to be back among my own people.
Song of Solomon 6:11-12 (TLB)

Lord, today I am feeling like this . . .

Mountaintops are for inspiration.
But it's in the **valley** where the **fruit grows**.

FEBRUARY 5

As the sun went down that evening,
all the villagers who had any sick people in their **homes,**
no matter what their diseases were,

brought them to Jesus;
and the **touch** of His hands **healed** every one!

Some were possessed by demons;
and the demons came out at His command, shouting,
"You are the Son of God."

But because they knew He was the Christ,
He stopped them and told them to be silent.

Luke 4:40-41 (TLB)

FEBRUARY 6

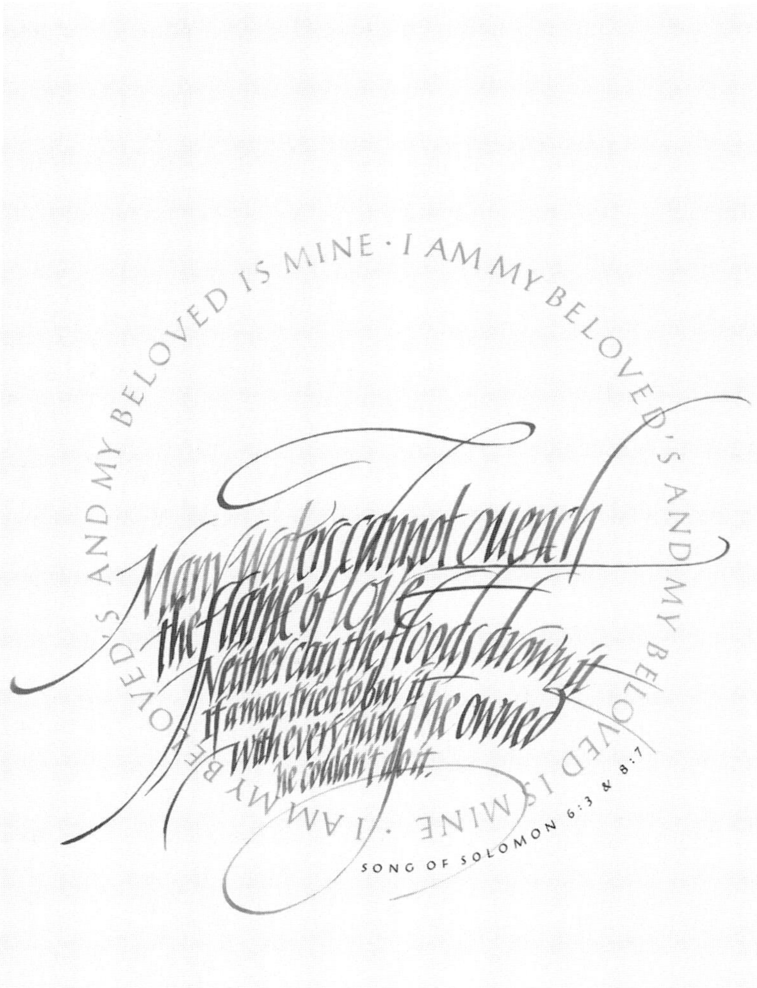
AND MY BELOVED IS MINE · I AM MY BELOVED'S AND MY BELOVED IS MINE · I AM MY BELOVED'S
Many waters cannot quench
the flame of love
Neither can the floods drown it
If a man tried to buy it
with everything he owned
he couldn't do it.
SONG OF SOLOMON 6:3 & 8:7

FEBRUARY 7

SAVED

Four arteries are blocked. One 100 percent and two 90 percent. Open heart surgery will be needed this week.

Medical tests are given. Results are analyzed. Decisions are made. Informational booklets and videos are given to the patient to explain the procedure. Tours are given to show surgery rooms, recovery room, and ICU rooms.

Tender words are shared from family to patient on the morning of surgery. Eyes meet and hold on, hands clasp and don't want to let go, prayers and kisses are shared, tears well up, and nervous small talk fills the waiting time until the point of no return.

Then the long wait begins for the family. There are visits with family and friends who haven't taken time to be together because of life's busy schedules. Let's get something to eat.

Surgery interrupts life's schedules. **S T O P!!**

The hospital is alive with multitudes of people in multicolored uniforms who each have a specific job to do and a gift to share in the common goal of making patients healthy.

High-tech, expensive equipment is utilized to make the patients well and whole again. People and technology are in synchronization for the common goal of **"s a v i n g"** patients' lives. At that point of no return, all technology and talent flow into action to return life to a body.

In wisdom and love, God has created a healthy, disciplined way of life and the free will to choose how one will live that life. He reaches out to **s a v e** us in all the stages of our life - and even at the emergency stage - the point of no return - He is there with His healing energy to **h e a l** us.

Written when Ron's brother had open heart surgery, February 9, 1989.

FEBRUARY 8

And God called the light **day**,
and the darkness He called **night**.
And there was evening and there was morning, **one day. . . .**

And God called the expanse **heaven**.
And there was evening and there was morning, a **second day. . . .**

And God called the dry land **earth**,
and the gathering of the waters He called **seas**;
        And God saw that it was good. . .
And the earth brought forth vegetation, . . .
        and God saw that it was good.
And there was evening and there was morning, a **third day. . . .**

Then God made the two great **lights**,
the greater light to govern the day,
and the lesser light to govern the night;
He made the stars also.
        And God saw that it was good.
And there was evening and there was morning, a **fourth day.**

And God said, "Let the waters teem with swarms of living creatures,
and let birds fly above the earth
in the open expanse of the heavens. . ."
        And God saw that is was good.
And there was evening and there was morning, a **fifth day. . . .**

And God made the **beasts** of the earth . . .
        and God saw that it was good.
And God created **man** in His own image,
in the image of God He created him;
male and female He created them. . . .
        And God saw . . . that . . . it was **very good.**
And there was evening and there was morning, a **sixth day.**

Continued on February 9

FEBRUARY 9

Thus the heavens and the earth were completed, and all their hosts.
And by the **seventh day**
God completed His work which He had done;
And He rested on the seventh day
from all His work which He had done.

Then God **blessed** the **seventh day** and sanctified it,
because **in it He rested from all His work**
which God had created and made.

Selected portions from Genesis 1:5-2:3 NAS

Creator God,

In Your creation process, the evening **darkness** came before the morning **light**. Create in me the awareness that morning light will illumine this time of darkness in my life.

Speak Your **order and peace** into my life as You did when You created everything. One day at a time - bring Your **light** into this darkness. Send Your Holy Spirit to hover over this chaotic situation.

I know that **spring always follows winter.** Lord, help my unbelief!

FEBRUARY 10

Rejoice in the Lord always;
Again I will say, rejoice!

Let your forbearing spirit be known to all men.
The Lord is near.

Be anxious for nothing,
but in everything by **prayer** and **supplication**
with **thanksgiving**
let your requests be made known to God.

And the **peace** of God,
which surpasses all comprehension,
shall guard your hearts and your minds in Christ Jesus.

Finally, brethren, whatever is

true honorable right
pure lovely good repute
if there is any excellence
if anything worthy of praise,

let your mind dwell on these things . . . .

And my God shall supply **all** your needs
according to His riches in glory in Christ Jesus.

Philippians 4:4-8, 19 NAS

FEBRUARY 11

Then God told him (Moses),

"**I will certainly be with you**,
and this is the proof that I am the one who is sending you:
When you have led the people out of Egypt,
you shall **worship** God here upon this **mountain**!"

Exodus 3:12 (TLB)

Lord, today I am feeling like this . . .

Don't forget in the valley
what you learned on the **mountaintop**.

FEBRUARY 12

LOVE is very patient and kind,
never jealous or envious,
never boastful or proud,
never haughty or selfish or rude.

LOVE does not demand its own way.

LOVE is not irritable or touchy.

LOVE does not hold grudges and
will hardly even notice when others do it wrong.

LOVE is never glad about injustice,
but rejoices whenever truth wins out.

If you LOVE someone
you will be loyal to him no matter what the cost.

You will always believe in him,
always expect the best of him, and
always stand your ground in defending him. . . .

There are three things that remain -

faith, hope, and love -

and the greatest of these is LOVE.

1 Corinthians 13:4-7, 13 (TLB)

FEBRUARY 13

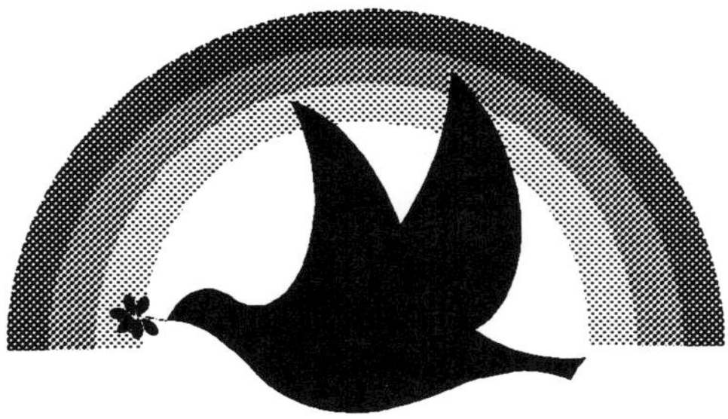

LOVE IS THE COLOR OF A RAINBOW

RED	flows from the heart
ORANGE	dependable as the sun
YELLOW	bright and warm
GREEN	grows
BLUE	calm
INDIGO	peaceful
VIOLET	passionate

Written February 14, 1979, our 20th Anniversary

FEBRUARY 14

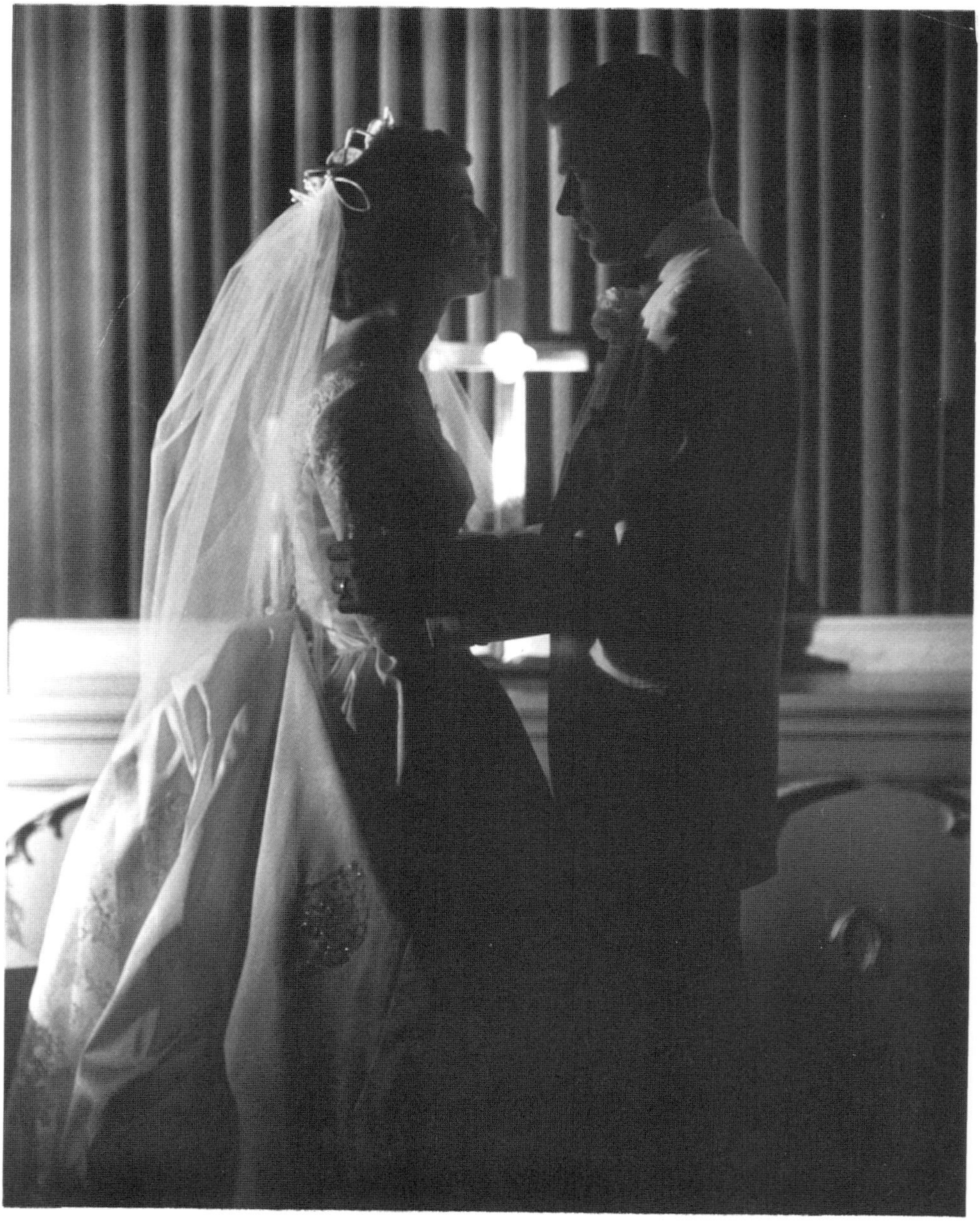

Our wedding picture, February 14, 1959
Ohmar Park Methodist Church, Dayton, Ohio

FEBRUARY 15

________________, will you have________________

to be your husband,
to live together in holy marriage?

Will you love him,
comfort him
honor and keep him,
in **sickness** and in **health**,
and forsaking all others,
be faithful to him
as long as you both shall live?

I will.

In the name of God,

I,________________, take you,________________

to be my husband,

to have and to hold
from this day forward,
for better, for worse,
for richer, for poorer,
sickness and in **health**,
to **love** and to **cherish**,
until we are parted by death.

This is my solemn vow.

FEBRUARY 16

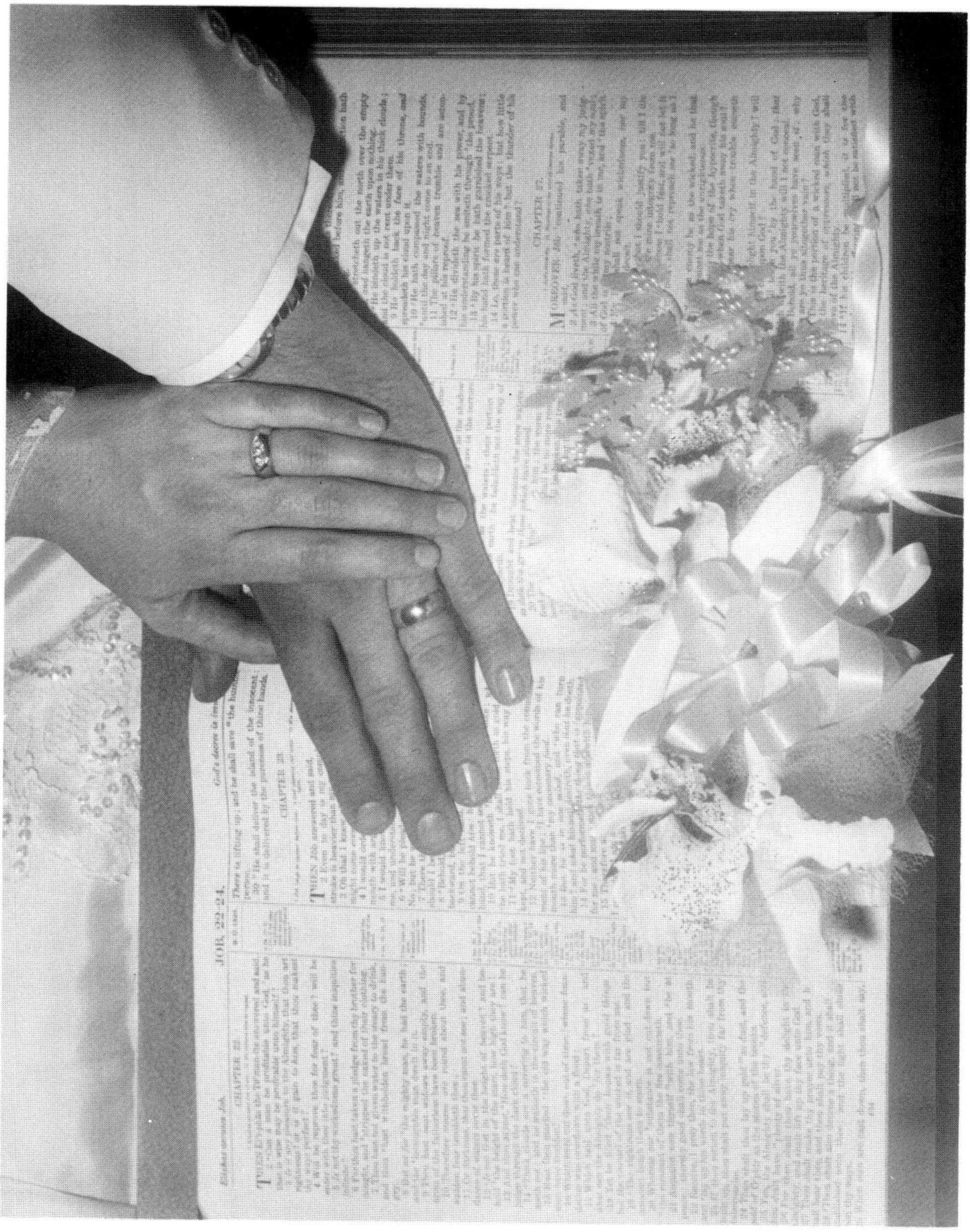

FEBRUARY 17

In our wedding album is my favorite picture of Ron and me. We are standing in silhouette before the altar cross. As I looked at it while preparing this devotional - for the first time ever - in 32 years - I **really** looked at the picture next to it.

Our hands are on a Bible. Then I looked closer at the passages in the Bible. **Job!!** Job 23:10 states: "But He (God) knows the way I take; When He has tried me, I shall come forth as gold."

I am sure the photographer had no idea what page in the Bible he opened to as he set the photograph. But God **knew**! Again God speaks to me, transcending time. He is refining me as gold. I am living on the food of His Word. I will not be silenced by this darkness in our life. I will continue to give God the Glory!!!

Look up in your Bible, Job 27:3-4 and write it out below.

____

____

Check out Job 23:12b. What does it say to you today?

____

____

What about Job 23:16-17. Is God speaking to you?

____

____

____

FEBRUARY 18

The King's daughter is all glorious within;

Her clothing is interwoven with gold.

Psalm 45:13 NAS

Lord, today I am feeling like this . . .

There's a golden thread woven in the pattern of my life's fabric, sewn by God, the Master Weaver.

FEBRUARY 19

As Jesus and the disciples were going to the rabbi's home,

a woman who had been sick for **twelve years**
with internal bleeding came up behind Him

and **touched** a tassel of His robe,

for she thought,

"If I only **touch Him**, I will be **healed**."

Jesus turned around and spoke to her.

"Daughter," He said, *"all is well!*
*Your **faith** has **healed** you."*

And the woman was well from that moment.

Matthew 9:19-22 (TLB). Also see Mark 5:25-34, Luke 8:43-48.

FEBRUARY 20

Celebrate!
Celebrate!
Celebrate!
Peanut Butter and Honey!

Today my soul is overflowing with peanut butter and honey!

Because - over this past year - through the

Great Experiment and the *Workbook of Living Prayer*
and the *Workbook of Intercessory Prayer*

God has taken the good soil of my life and
cleaned out the rocks and weeds.

Now my soul is prepared for new growth.

In Ezekiel 2 and 3, the Lord says:

"Open Your Mouth
Feed on My Word
Get Filled Up With My Words"

Then I ate it, and it **was** sweet as honey in my mouth!
During my physical craving for peanut butter and honey,
My soul has hungered to be fed
And God has fed me a **banquet**
Overflowing with the best treats He has.

Now my soul is ready to reproduce the fruits of
God's Love and Spirit and to invite **all** to the Banquet Table.

Oh! come, taste and see that the Lord is Good!

Salt! Lord! Salt!

Now I **see**! Salt makes me thirsty for the **living water**.

Oh! Come, taste, and see that the Lord is Good!

Written February 20, 1988

FEBRUARY 21

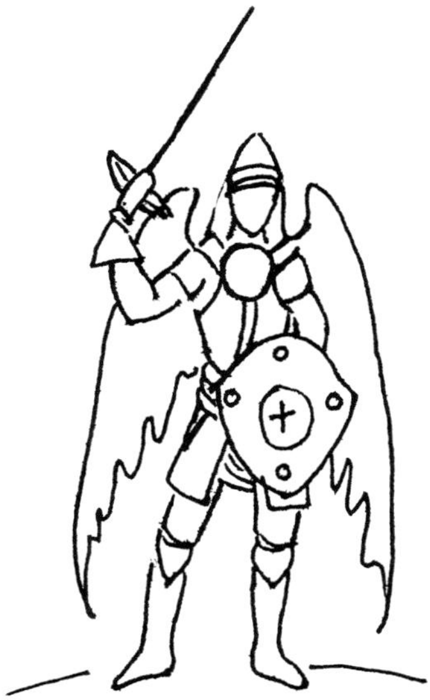

PROTECTING ANGELS

My God sent His angel and shut the lions' mouths, and
they have not harmed me . . . Daniel 6:22 NAS

RESCUE ANGELS

In all their distress He too was distressed, and
the angel of His presence saved them.
In His love and mercy He redeemed them;
He lifted them up and carried them . . . Isaiah 63:9 NIV

MESSENGER ANGELS

But after he had considered this, an angel of the Lord appeared to him in a dream and said, "Joseph son of David, do not be afraid to take Mary home as your wife, because what is conceived in her is from the Holy Spirit."

Matthew 1:20 NIV

FEBRUARY 22

LOST

Flight 838 from Chicago to Columbus was due to arrive at 10:34 P.M. When it had not arrived by 11:00, we went looking for someone who might have information about the flight. No one was available at that time of night. About 11:10 the plane came in.

We watched as the passengers disembarked. Businessmen with brief cases hurrying home after a long day . . . beauticians returning from a convention . . . families embracing . . . but **no** Betsy, our daughter. We looked at each other in confusion. "She's sick," flashed through my mind, because she had been earlier in the week. Down the enclosed walkway I went toward the plane to see if she was there. "No passengers left on board," assured the leaving stewardess and pilots.

The flight attendant looked on the computer. The originating flight from Kansas City was 2 1/2 hours late. "She's rescheduled for 6:00 A.M. tomorrow," she said.

We looked at each other, questioning this information. She had been sick. Is she OK? Where will she stay tonight? She had no car at the Kansas City airport. How will she make a rescheduled 6:00 A.M. flight?

No one was available in the terminal at 11:30 P.M. to do further checking. Should we go back home? . . . a two-hour drive because of snow squalls.

We called our son, Steve, in Kansas City. No, he had not heard anything. No she had not gone to her apartment. Kansas City airport said the original flight finally left but was redirected to Milwaukee.

What to do at midnight? Where is she? Sleeping on the Kansas City airport floor? Is she OK?

A call to an 800 number for the airline repeated the earlier message that she was rescheduled for a morning flight, but could offer no proof of where she was overnight.

Continued on February 23

FEBRUARY 23

"So, you are telling me to **trust** the message that she will be on the 6:00 A.M. flight?"

"Yes."

The two-hour ride home begins at midnight.

Awakening at 7:15 A.M., my first thought is - call the airline to verify if she did, in fact, board the 6:00 A.M. flight in Kansas City.

"Can't release that information and it wouldn't be available yet." The operator transferred the call. I repeat the story.

"Yes, she's on that flight!"

Praise the Lord! Knowing brings relief. My morning devotional uses the scripture found in 1 John 4:18 ". . . love casts out fear. . . "

I was overwhelmed by the realization that the fear, concern, and questions of where our loved one was physically, and the frustration of not being able to communicate with her, are like the emotions of having a loved one **"lost"** spiritually. Expecting them **"home."** The frustration and concern of not knowing where they are. Reaching out to others for help in finding them. The final realization. **Trust**.

Go Home. Sleep. **Trust.**

Then the **joy** of a morning call!!!

"Mom! I made the flight, I'm in Dallas, awaiting the flight to Columbus. Tell you all about it when I get there!!"

Praise the Lord!! The **joy** of being reunited!!

And the **joy** of spiritual insight when it dawns in loved ones. The knowing look in their eyes as the confusion leaves and **truth** lights up their eyes.

Welcome home!! The **joy** of reunited spirits!!

Written February 11, 1989

FEBRUARY 24

But if we must keep trusting God

for something that hasn't happened yet,

it teaches us to wait **patiently** and confidently.

Romans 8:25 (TLB)

Lord, today I am feeling like this . . .

Patience is the ability to keep your motor idling
when you feel like stripping your gears.

FEBRUARY 25

In January of 1988 we were asked to be facilitators for a video marriage enrichment series called *Teammates*. Through this experience I learned so much about myself and others and how to appreciate everyone's strengths and work with their weaknesses.

As I became a Caregiver, I realized a new use for this information. God prepared me so that I would know my strengths and weaknesses in this new role. I also needed to know Ron's strengths and weaknesses and how he functioned and thought as God created him.

Putting this information into practice eased some of the daily tension, confusion, and anxiety of caregiving.

On the following two pages are listed the strengths and weaknesess of four different temperaments. See if you can find yourself and also the others in your family or friends. You may find that you are a combination of several temperaments.

Then ask God to show you how to incorporate this knowledge into your daily life. Ask Him to show you how to love your loved ones in light of their temperament.

The February 28th devotional is intercessory prayer Scriptures for each temperament and a place for you to insert the names for whom you are praying. Each temperament needs different prayer.

The Holy Spirit showed me the meaning of the first letters of the temperaments:

D oer
I nfluencer
R elator
T hinker

DIRT. DIRT? DIRT! Genesis 2:7 "Then the Lord God formed man of dust from the ground, and breathed into his nostrils the breath of life; and man became a living being."

See Works Cited Page for additional information about the distribution of *Teammates*.

FEBRUARY 26

THE DOER

STRENGTHS

The ideal environment includes:

___Many new and varied activities
___Opportunity to get things done
___Continual challenges
___Difficult assignments
___Freedom to act
___Control over situations
___Direct answers from others

Tendencies include:

___Getting immediate results
___Making quick decisions
___Persistence
___Solving problems
___Taking charge
___Self-reliance
___Accepting challenges

WEAKNESSES

May have tendencies which include:

___Insensitivity to others
___Impatience
___Overlooks risks and cautions
___Inflexibility and unyielding
___Taking on too much
___Being inattentive to detail
___Resenting restrictions
___Being too demanding of others

Needs others to provide:

___Sensitivity to needs of others
___Caution
___Details and facts

Has opportunities to trust God for:

___Patience
___Sensitivity to the needs of others
___Being more flexible

THE INFLUENCER

STRENGTHS

The ideal environment includes:

___A friendly atmosphere
___Freedom from control and detail
___Opportunity to influence others
___Public recognition of ability
___Opportunity to verbalize
___Positive reinforcement and praise
___Enthusiastic response to ideas

Tendencies include:

___Optimism
___Enthusiasm
___Being personable
___Making a good impression
___Being verbally articulate
___A desire to help others
___Creating an entertaining climate

WEAKNESSES

May have tendencies which include:

___Lack of follow-through
___Over-selling
___Over-estimating anticipated results
___Misjudging capabilities
___Talking too much
___Acting Impulsively
___Jumping to conclusions
___Over-committing

Needs others to provide

___Follow-through on detail
___A logical approach
___Concentration on the task

Has opportunities to trust God

___Better control of time
___Objectivity in decision making
___Pausing before acting

FEBRUARY 27

THE RELATER

STRENGTHS

The ideal environment includes:

___Sincere appreciation
___Minimal conflict
___Security
___Acknowledgement of work
___Limited territory
___Opportunity to develop relationships
___Traditional way of doing things

Tendencies include:

___Being supportive
___Being agreeable
___Loyalty
___Self-control
___Consistency
___Being a good listener
___Performing established work patterns

WEAKNESSES

May have tendencies which include:

___Resisting change
___Trouble meeting deadlines
___Being overly lenient
___Procrastinating
___Being indecisive
___Holding a grudge
___Being overly possessive
___Lack of initiative

Needs others to provide:

___Stretch toward challenge
___Help in solving difficult problems
___Initiative and change

Has opportunities to trust God for:

___Facing confrontation
___Initiating more
___Increasing pace

THE THINKER

STRENGTHS

The ideal environment includes:

___Being able to concentrate on detail
___Opportunities to critique
___Stable surroundings
___Opportunities for reassurance
___An exact job description
___Opportunities for careful planning
___Time to do things right

Tendencies include:

___Orderliness
___Conscientiousness
___Discipline
___Preciseness
___Thoroughness
___Being diplomatic with people
___Being analytical

WEAKNESSES

May have tendencies which include:

___Indecisiveness
___Getting bogged down in detail
___Rigidness of the how to
___Overly avoiding conflict
___Low self-esteem
___Being hesitant to try new things
___Resisting full responsibility
___Pessimism

Needs others to provide:

___Quick decision making
___Reassurance
___Stretching of capabilities

Has opportunities to trust God

___Being more open
___Self-confidence
___Being more optimistic

FEBRUARY 28

INTERCESSORY PRAYER SCRIPTURES

FOR DOERS

________will hear and increase in learning, ________will be a person of understanding and ________will acquire wise counsel. Proverbs 1:5 NAS

The way of ________is right in ________own eyes, but ________listens to counsel. Proverbs 12:15 NAS

This ________knows. Be quick to hear, slow to speak, and slow to anger.
James 1:19 NAS

FOR INFLUENCERS

Therefore if ________is in Christ, ________is a new creature; the old things passed away; new things have come. 2 Corinthians 5:17 NAS

Don't talk so much. ________keeps putting your foot in your mouth. Be sensible and turn off the flow! Proverbs 10:19 (TLB)

Be sure that everything is done properly in a good and orderly way.
1 Corinthians 14:40 (TLB)

FOR RELATORS

Open rebuke is better than hidden love! Proverbs 27:5 (TLB)

Now an angel from heaven appeared to ________, strengthening ________.
Luke 22:43 NAS

Be wise, make use of every opportunity ________has for doing good.
Ephesians 5:16 (TLB)

FOR THINKERS

For God has not given ________a spirit of timidity, but of power and love and discipline. 2 Timothy 1:7 NAS

Devote ________ to prayer, keeping ________alert in it with an attitude of thanksgiving; praying at the same time for _________ as well, that God may open up to _______ a door for the word, so that ________ may speak forth the mystery of Christ . . . Colossians 4:2-3 NAS

MARCH 1

So Jesus climbed into a boat and went across the lake to
Capernaum, His home town.

Soon some men brought Him a paralyzed boy on a mat.

When Jesus saw **their faith**, He said to the sick boy,

"Cheer up, son! For I have forgiven your sins!"

"Blasphemy! This man is saying He is God!"
exclaimed some of the religious leaders to themselves.

Jesus knew what they were thinking and asked them,

"Why are you thinking such evil thoughts?
I, the Messiah, have the authority on earth to forgive sins.
But talk is cheap - anybody could say that.
So I'll prove it to you by healing this man."

Then, turning to the paralyzed man, He commanded,

"Pick up you stretcher and go on home,
for you are healed."

And the boy jumped up and left!

A chill of fear swept through the crowd as they saw this happen right before their eyes. How they praised God for giving such authority to a man!

Matthew 9:1-8 (TLB). Also see Mark 2:3-12.

MARCH 2

Then the LORD spoke to Moses, saying,

"Speak to Aaron and to his sons, saying,

'Thus you shall bless the sons of Israel.
You shall say to them:

The LORD bless you, and keep you;
The LORD make His face shine on you,
And be gracious to you;
The LORD lift up His countenance on you,
And give you peace.'

"So they shall invoke **My name** on the sons of Israel, and

I then will bless them."

Numbers 6:22-27 NAS

God of all **blessings**, I will learn to **speak in love,**
this **blessing** to my loved one as You commanded Aaron
to do. I praise You for the blessing of Your presence **with** us.

MARCH 3

And let us not lose heart in doing good,

for in due time we shall reap

if we do not grow weary.

Galatians 6:9 NAS

Lord, today I am feeling like this . . .

MARCH 4

Yet those who **wait** for the LORD will gain new strength;
They will mount up with wings like eagles,
They will run and not get tired,
They will walk and not become weary. Isaiah 40:31 NAS

Silence is not the absence of sound, but the presence of God. In today's sound-saturated world, it is difficult to find silence. Distracting sounds surround me and deaden my ears to God's voice.

It requires a concentrated effort to take time to be **holy**. Brakes have to be applied to my life so that I can wait upon the Lord. I can say sentence prayers about the events and needs during the day. But I have to **take** time to be holy and **wait** upon the Lord. That's when God speaks to me. That's when I am not weary.

I do get bogged down and weary when I fail to practice the presence of God.

God of rest and quiet places, You do speak to me when I wait upon You. Teach me, Lord, how to wait when the demands of the day overtake me. Bring stillness to my soul. Meet me in those quiet moments with Your peace.

Written for a Lenten Devotional, 1986

MARCH 5

. . . the rabbi of the local synagogue came and **worshiped** Him.

> "My little daughter has just died," he said,
> but You can bring her back to life again
> if You will only come and **touch** her." . . .

When Jesus arrived at the rabbi's home and saw the noisy crowds and heard the funeral music, He said,

> *"Get them out,*
> *for the little girl isn't dead;*
> *she is only sleeping!"*

Then how they all scoffed and sneered at Him!

When the crowd was finally outside,
Jesus went in where the little girl was lying
and took her by the hand,
and she jumped up
and was all right again!

The report of this wonderful miracle swept the entire countryside.

Matthew 9:18, 23-26 (TLB). Also see Mark 5:22, 35-42, Luke 8:41, 49-56.

MARCH 6

PASTOR'S ICE PRAYER

Lord, as we beheld the after-effects of this week's winter storm,
and saw dead limbs fallen from trees, and even live ones,
crushed by the weight of ice,
driven to the ground by the force of the wind,
we were reminded again of the debris in our lives,
For we have responded to cold hearts and cold shoulders
with icy unforgiveness,
and sometimes hunks of our relationships lie fallen in ruin before us.

Lord, we regret the storms and their after-effects in our relationships.
We pray that when they come,
You will forgive us and enable us to overcome them.

As the green growth of trees is enhanced by nature's pruning of dead limbs,
so may the stormy times enhance the green growth of our relationships.
Through our separations may we evaluate what went wrong, and
open ourselves to be transformed for new life that finds itself free to grow.

As good but injured limbs eventually heal,
so may the wounds in our relationships not last forever,
but eventually grow together into tissues of new life,
leaving us in one piece and ready to relate again.

And Lord, as we do not leave nature's debris lying around
to clutter up our sidewalks and streets,
so may You cleanse our hearts of dead hunks of the past.
You were wounded for our transgressions, Your Word tells us.
You were bruised for our iniquities. With Your stripes we are healed.
Heal us, then, Lord. Do not let Your death for us be in vain.
By our forgiveness of one another, take away the after-effects of our wrongs.

And Lord, even as the sun comes out to melt the ice at last,
before it can destroy the trees entirely,
so come to us in Your Son Jesus, and melt the hardness of our heart
through the emotional and spiritual warmth of His love.

With Your power-lines that never fail, convert our ice into streams of living water, reconciling and renewing our relationships in His name.

AMEN.

Bob Campbell, Greenfield, Ohio March 6, 1988

MARCH 7

SPRING ALWAYS FOLLOWS WINTER

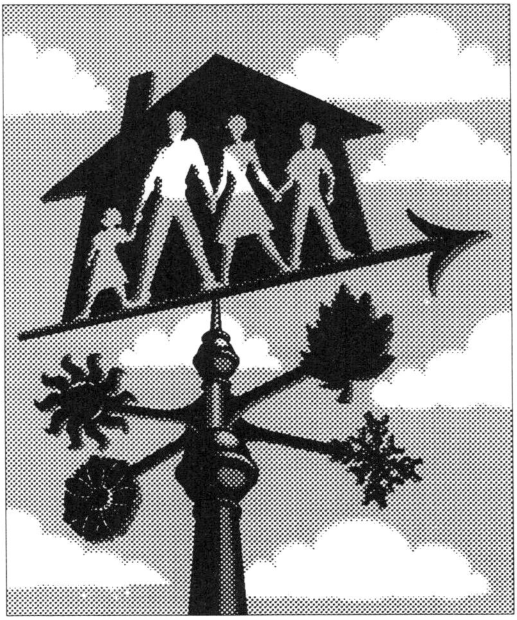

For there is hope for a tree, when it is cut down,
that it will sprout again, and its shoots will not fail.
Though its roots grow old in the ground,
and its stump dies in the dry soil,

at the scent of water

it will flourish and put forth sprigs like a plant.

Job 14:7-9 NAS

MARCH 8

David therefore inquired of God for the child;
and David fasted and went and lay all night on the ground.

And the elders of his household stood beside him
in order to raise him up from the ground,
but he was unwilling and
would not eat food with them.

Then it happened on the seventh day that the **child died**.
And the servants of David were afraid to tell him
that the child was dead, for they said,

"Behold, while the child was still alive,
we spoke to him and he did not listen to our voice.
How then can we tell him that the child is dead,
since he might do himself harm!"

But when David saw that his servants were whispering together,
David perceived that the child was dead;
so David said to his servants,

"Is the child dead?"

And they said, "He is dead."

So David **arose** from the ground, **washed**,
anointed himself, and **changed** his clothes;
and he came into the house of the LORD
and **worshiped**.

Then he came to his own house,
and when he requested,
they set food before him and he **ate**.

Continued on March 9

MARCH 9

WISDOM BORN OUT OF GRIEF

Then his servants said to him,

"What is this thing that you have done?
While the child was alive, you fasted and wept;
but when the child died, you arose and ate food."

And he said,

"While the child was still alive, I fasted and wept;
for I said,
'Who knows, the LORD may be gracious to me,
that the child may live.'
"But now he has died; why should I fast?
Can I bring him back again?
I shall go to him, but he will not return to me."

Then David comforted his wife Bathsheba,
and went in to her and lay with her;
and she gave birth to a son,
and he named him Solomon.
Now the Lord loved him . . .

2 Samuel 12:16-24 NAS

MARCH 10

If Thy law had not been my delight,

Then I would have perished in my affliction.

Psalm 119:92 NAS

Lord, today I am feeling like this . . .

MARCH 11

Be gracious to me, O LORD,
        for I am pining away;
Heal me, O LORD,
        for my bones are dismayed.
And my soul is greatly dismayed;
        But Thou, O LORD - how long?

Return, O LORD, rescue my soul;
        Save me because of Thy lovingkindness.
For there is no mention of Thee in death;
        In Sheol who will give Thee thanks?

I am weary with my sighing;
        Every night I make my bed swim,
                I dissolve my couch with my tears.
My eye has wasted away with grief;
        It has become old because of all my adversaries.

Depart from me, all you who do iniquity,
        For the LORD has heard the voice of my weeping.
The LORD has heard my supplication,
        The LORD receives my prayer.

All my enemies shall be ashamed and greatly dismayed;
        They shall turn back,
                they shall suddenly be ashamed.

Psalm 6:2-10 NAS

MARCH 12

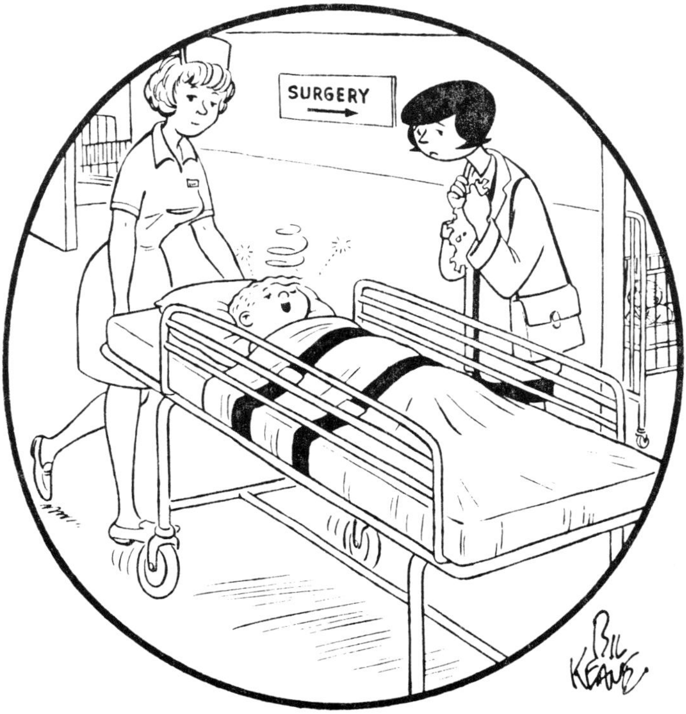

"I won't get hurt, Mommy, they fastened my seat belts."

MARCH 13

Then the King will say to those on His right,

'Come, you who are blessed of My Father,
inherit the kingdom prepared for you
from the foundation of the world.

For I was **hungry** . . .	you gave Me something to **eat**
I was **thirsty** . . .	you gave Me **drink**
I was **a stranger** . . .	you **invited** Me in
I was **naked** . . .	you **clothed** Me
I was **sick** . . .	you **visited** Me
I was **in prison** . .	you **came** to Me.'

Then the righteous will answer Him, saying,

'Lord, when did we see You hungry, thirsty, a stranger, naked, sick, or in prison . . .?'

And the King will answer and say to them,

'Truly I say to you,
to the extent that you did it
to one of these brothers of Mine,
even the least of them,
you did it to Me.'

Matthew 25:34-40 NAS

MARCH 14

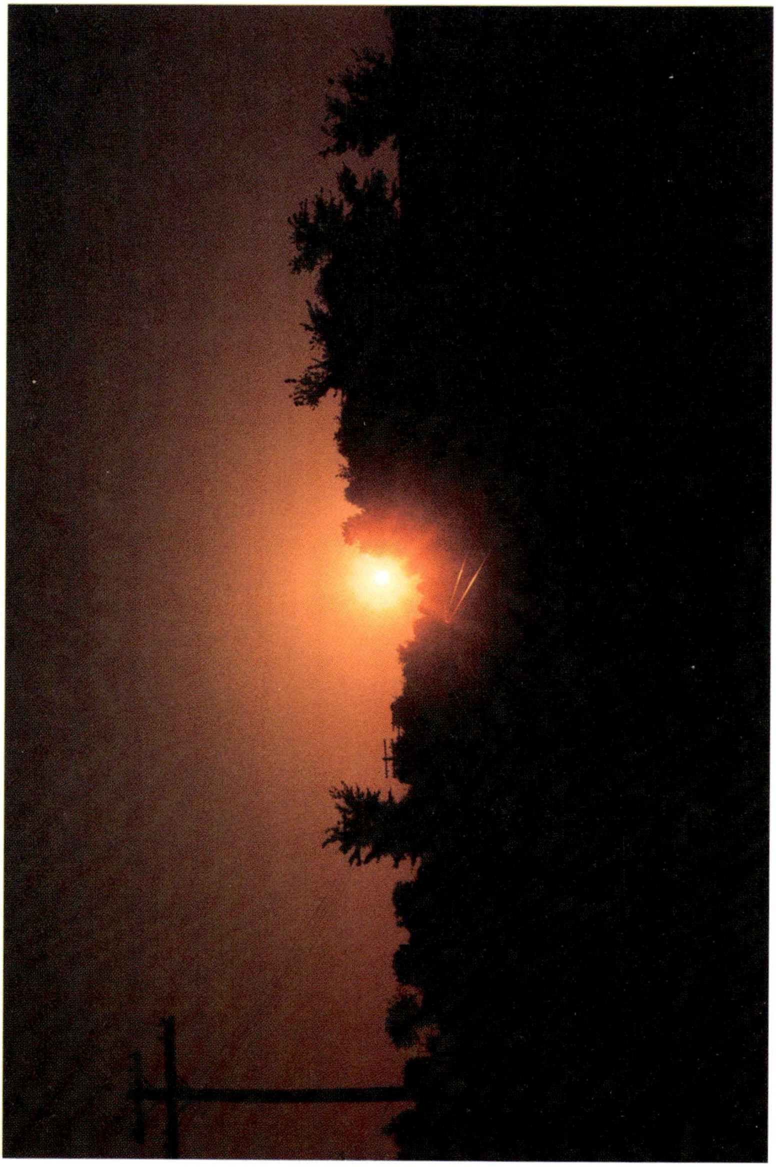

Photograph by Sharon Sims

MARCH 15

During the winter and spring months of 1990, we were going to many different doctors for testing and diagnosis for Ron's illness. At that time a friend showed me a series of pictures she had taken outside our town of Greenfield, Ohio.

WOW!! This picture captivated me!!

Immediately, **light in my darkness**, came to me.

See the railroad tracks? They curve into the unknown but also into the **light**. God's Light is there waiting to guide me on my unknown path . . . if I stay on the tracks.

See, also, the three telephone poles? They speak to me of receiving messages from God . . . if I **listen** to Him.

The day after I first saw this picture, The Holy Spirit gave me Psalm 27 - and I **knew** He was speaking to me about allowing Him to be the **light in my darkness.**

The Lord is my **light** and my **salvation**;
whom shall I fear?

The one thing I want from God, the thing I seek most of all,
is the privilege of meditating in His Temple,
living in His presence every day of my life,
delighting in His incomparable perfections and glory.

There I'll be when troubles come. He will hide me.
He will set me on a high rock out of reach of all my enemies.
Then I will bring Him sacrifices and sing His praises with much joy.

Psalm 27:1, 4-7 (TLB)

MARCH 16

One Sabbath as He was teaching in a synagogue,
He saw a seriously handicapped woman
who had been bent double for **eighteen years**
and was unable to straighten herself.

Calling her over to Him Jesus said,

*"Woman, you are **healed** of your sickness!"*

He **touched** her, and **instantly** she could stand straight.
How she praised and thanked God!

Luke 13:10-13 (TLB)

MARCH 17

I weep with grief;

my heart is heavy with sorrow;

encourage and cheer me with Your words.

Psalm 119:28 (TLB)

Lord, today I am feeling like this . . .

Gaining insight is like an onion,
peeling off layers of skin
and crying a little.

MARCH 18

But He knows the way I take;

when He has tried me,

I shall come forth as gold.

My foot has held fast to His path;

I have kept His way and

not turned aside.

I have not departed from the command of His lips;

I have treasured the words of His mouth

more than my necessary food.

Job 23:10-12 NAS

MARCH 19

WAIT

Moses	40 days on Mt. Sinai being instructed by God in the Law
Israelites	40 years wandering in the desert
Noah	40 days of rain
Sarah	90 years old when first child was born
Jesus	30 years living and working at home
Jesus	40 days in desert before beginning His ministry
Jesus	3 days in tomb
Disciples	waiting in the Upper Room for the Holy Spirit

Waiting rooms in your life

Doctors, Accountants, Boss, Lawyers, Principals, Hospital, Surgery

Waiting times in your life

Birth of a child, rains to end, spring's first flower, tomatoes to ripen, Christmas to come, graduation day, wedding day, prodigal to return, healing, coming of Jesus

And gathering them together, He (Jesus) commanded them not to leave Jerusalem, but to **wait** for what the Father had promised . . . you shall receive **power** when the Holy Spirit has come upon you; and you shall be My witnesses both in Jerusalem, and in all Judea and Samaria, and even to the remotest part of the earth.

Acts 1:4,8 NAS

MARCH 20

PRAYER FOR CAREGIVERS

May the LORD answer you when you are in distress;
may the name of the God of Jacob protect you.
May he send you help from the sanctuary
and grant you support from Zion.

May he remember all your sacrifices
and accept your burnt offerings.
May he give you the desire of your heart
and make all your plans succeed.

We will shout for joy when you are victorious
and will lift up our banners in the name of our God.

May the LORD grant all your requests.
Now I know that the LORD saves his anointed;
he answers him from his holy heaven
with the saving power of his right hand.

Some trust in chariots and some in horses,
but **we trust in the name of the LORD our God.**
They are brought to their knees and fall,
but we rise up and stand firm.

O LORD, save the king!
Answer us when we call!

Psalm 20 NIV

MARCH 21

Is anyone among you **suffering**?
Let **him pray**.
Is anyone **cheerful**?
Let **him sing praises**.
Is anyone among you **sick**?
Let **him call** for the elders of the church,
and let **them pray** over him,
anointing him with **oil**
in the name of the Lord;
and **the prayer offered in faith**
will **restore** the one who is sick,
and the Lord will raise him up,
and if he has committed sins,
they will be forgiven him.

Therefore, **confess** your sins to one another,
and **pray** for one another,
so that you may be healed.

The effective prayer of a righteous man
can accomplish much.

James 5:13-16 NAS

God of healing, I pray for this one who is in need of Your healing touch.
Prayers for the physical healing of this body.
Prayers for wisdom of the doctors.
Prayers for the medicine to fulfill its purpose in this body.
Prayers for the Holy Spirit to raise up the sins that need to be confessed.
Prayers for Your will to be done and for the peace of heart to accept Your will.
I wait before You as You work Your will. Your Grace, Mercy, Peace and Love flow with healing through this body, mind, and soul.
I praise You and give You the glory for what You are doing in this body and in this life.

MARCH 22

WOMAN'S ECCLESIASTES

There is a right time for everything in a woman's life,

A time to smile
A time to cry,

A time to study
A time to goof off,

A time to giggle
A time to be serious,

A time to be a student
A time to be an employee,

A time to question
A time to know God,

A time to be an athlete
A time to be a spectator.

A time to be a friend
A time to be a lover,

A time to live alone
A time to marry,

A time to give birth
A time to nurture,

A time to stay home
A time to volunteer,

A time to be sick
A time to nurse.

A time to be frantic
A time to be relaxed,

A time to create
A time to observe

A time to chauffeur
A time to walk,

A time to eat desserts
A time to diet,

A time to hold tight
A time to let go,

A time to worry
A time to pray.

A time to be a club member
A time to hold an office,

A time to receive help
A time to serve others,

A time to read
A time to listen,

A time to cook
A time to eat out,

A time to look back
and remember,

Everything is appropriate in its own time.
Woman cannot see the whole scope of God's work from beginning to end.
She must appreciate and enjoy each time she is in and
look forward to the new adventures God has in store for her.

Written in 1978 when my first son graduated from high school

MARCH 23

And now the blind and crippled came to Him
and He **healed** them there in the Temple.

But when the chief priests and other Jewish leaders
saw these wonderful miracles,
and heard even the little children in the Temple shouting,

"God bless the Son of David,"

they were disturbed and indignant and asked Him,

"Do You hear what these children are saying?"

"Yes," Jesus replied.
"Didn't you ever read the Scriptures?
For they say, 'Even little babies shall praise Him!' "

On Monday of Holy Week

Matthew 21:14-16 (TLB). See also Psalm 8:2.

MARCH 24

So Joshua and his men went out to fight the army of Amalek. Meanwhile Moses, Aaron, and Hur went to the top of the hill. And as long as Moses held up the rod in his hands, Israel was winning; but whenever he rested his arms at his sides, the soldiers of Amalek were winning. Moses' arms finally became too tired to hold up the rod any longer; so Aaron and Hur rolled a stone for him to sit on, and they stood on each side, holding his hands until sunset.

Exodus 17:10-12 (TLB)

Lord, today I am feeling like this . . .

Big Bear Hugs from those who support me encourage me to **keep on keeping on**.

MARCH 25

Show me Your ways, O LORD,
teach me Your paths;
Guide me in Your truth and teach me,
for You are God my Savior,
and my **hope** is in You all day long.

Remember, O LORD, Your great mercy and love,
for they are from of old.
Remember not the sins of my youth and my rebellious ways;
according to Your love remember me,
for You are good, O LORD. . . .

Turn to me and be gracious to me,
for I am lonely and afflicted.
The troubles of my heart have multiplied;
free me from my anguish.
Look upon my affliction and my distress
and take away all my sins.

See how my enemies have increased and
and how fiercely they hate me!
Guard my life and rescue me;
let me not be put to shame,
for I take refuge in you.

May integrity and uprightness protect me, because

MY HOPE IS IN YOU.

Psalm 25:4-7, 16-21 NIV

MARCH 26

But He was pierced for our transgressions,
He was crushed for our iniquities;
the punishment that brought us peace was upon Him,
and **by His wounds we are healed.**

Isaiah 53:5 NIV

He Himself bore our sins in this body on the tree,
so that we might die to sins
and live for righteousness;
by His wounds you have been healed.

1 Peter 2:24 NIV

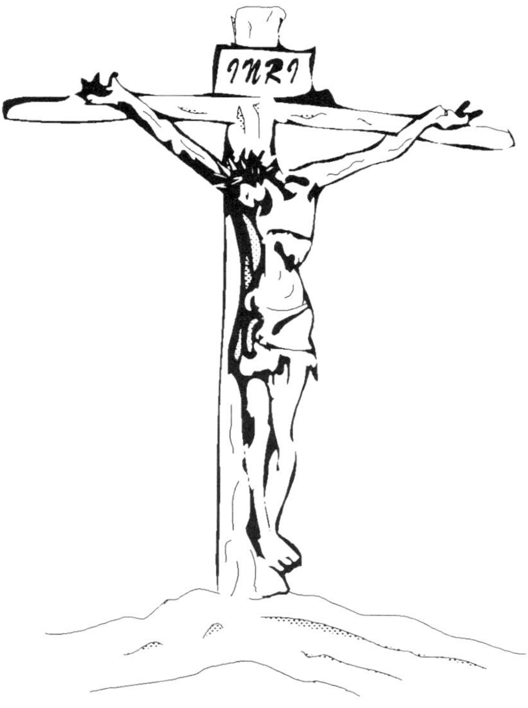

MARCH 27

HE LIVES

I serve a risen Savior, He's in the world today;
I know that He is living, whatever foes may say.
I see His hand of mercy, I hear His voice of cheer,
And just the time I need him, He's always near.

In all the world around me I see His loving care,
And though my heart grows weary, I never will despair.
I know that He is leading through all the stormy blast;
The day of His appearing will come at last.

Rejoice, rejoice, O Christian, lift up your voice and sing
Eternal hallelujahs to Jesus Christ the King!
The hope of all who seek Him the help of all who find;
None other is so loving, so good and kind.

He lives, He lives, Christ Jesus lives today!

He walks with me and talks with me along life's narrow way.

He lives, He lives, salvation to impart!

You ask me how I know He lives?

He lives within my heart.

Words and music by Alfred H. Ackley

MARCH 28

If you love Me, Obey Me;
and I will ask the Father
and He will give you
another **Comforter**,
and He will **never leave** you.

He is the *Holy Spirit*,
the Spirit who leads into all **truth**.

John 14:15-17 (TLB)

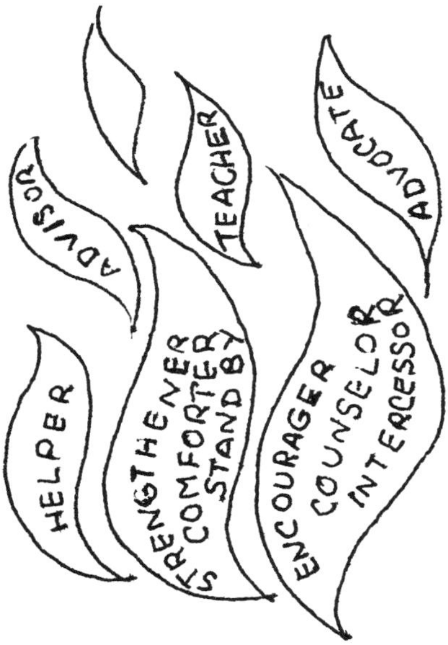

MARCH 29

Leaving that place,

Jesus met a man who couldn't speak
because a demon was inside him.

So Jesus cast out the demon,
and **instantly** the man could talk.

How the crowds marveled!

"Never in all our lives have we seen anything like this,"
they exclaimed.

Matthew 9:32-33 (TLB). See also Luke 11:14.

MARCH 30

You are the **light** of the world.
A city set on a hill cannot be hidden.
Nor do men light a lamp,
and put it under the peck measure,
but on the lamp stand;
and it **gives light** to all who are in the **house.**

Let **your light** shine before men in such a way
that they may **see** your good works,
and glorify your Father who is in heaven.
Matthew 5:14-16 NAS

Lord, today I am feeling like this . . .

I don't have to light all the world,
But I do have to light my part of it.

MARCH 31

CONFESSION

My kitchen table is in front of a window that looks out on a large bush where I have had a bird seed bell sitting all winter. When we are having our meals, we watch a pair of cardinals come for seeds. The other day the seed bell fell over and lodged on its side.

This morning I awoke to a beautiful snow. The delicate branches of the bush are piled high with fluffy snow. The overturned seed bell has over six inches of snow on it. But underneath - the seeds are still exposed for the cardinal's breakfast. I am now glad I didn't go and set up the bell. God is using something that is out of place to provide for His creation.

As I watch the beautiful bright red cardinals against the white snow, Scriptures come to mind. In the concordance I look up "snow" and find two appropriate verses. Psalm 51:7 says

" . . . wash me, and I shall be whiter than snow . . . . "

In Isaiah 1:18, the Lord says "Come now, and let us reason together, . . . Though your sins are as scarlet, they will be white as snow."

I realize that God has given me a message. I have to come together with other believers to share our faith. Even though things I have done stick out like a bright red cardinal, God provides daily for my needs and washes me clean as new fallen snow.

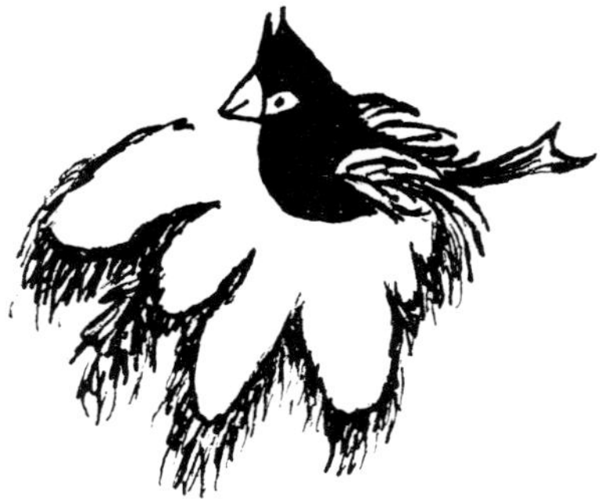

Written during the time of a broken relationship with a friend, and during the Great Experiment, March 31, 1987.

APRIL 1

When I kept silent about my sin,
my body wasted away
Through my groaning all day long.
For day and night Thy hand was heavy upon me;
My vitality was drained away as with the
fever heat of summer.

I acknowledged my sin to Thee,
And my iniquity I did not hide;
I said, "I will confess my transgression to the Lord";
And Thou didst forgive the guilt of my sin. . . .

Thou art my **hiding place;**
Thou dost preserve me from trouble;
Thou dost surround me with songs of deliverance.

I will **instruct** you and
teach you in the way which you should go;
I will **counsel** you with My eye upon you. . . .

Be glad in the Lord and rejoice you righteous ones,
And **shout for joy** all you who are upright in heart.

Psalm 32:3-5, 7-8, 11 NAS

APRIL 2

NOT **B I T T E R**

I = **S I N** - Selfish pity party

BUT **B E T T E R**

E = **E mmanuel** - God **with** me

Even though I **walk through**
the valley of the shadow of death,
I fear no evil;
For Thou art **with** me . . .

Psalm 23:4 NAS

APRIL 3

Jesus started to indicate to his disciples that he must go to Jerusalem and suffer greatly there. Matthew 16:21

Jesus faces his suffering and death directly, and he asks his disciples to face theirs the same way. He does not predict an easy future for himself or his disciples. Jesus went against the human inclination to avoid suffering and death, but his followers realized it was better to face up to the truth.

Suffering and death belong to the narrow road of Jesus. Jesus does not glorify them, or call them beautiful, good or something to be desired. Jesus does not call for heroism or suicidal self-sacrifice. No, Jesus invites us to look at the reality of our existence and reveals this harsh reality as the way to new life.

The core message of Jesus is that joy and peace can never be reached by bypassing suffering and death, but only by going right through them.

We can deny the reality of life or we can face it. When we face it with the eyes of Jesus, we discover that where we least expect it, something is hidden that holds a promise stronger than death itself. Jesus lived his life with the trust that God's love is stronger than death and that death therefore does not have the last word.

APRIL 4

And because of the surpassing greatness of the revelations,
for this reason,
to keep me from exalting myself,
there was given me a **thorn** in the **flesh**,
a messenger of Satan to buffet me -
to keep me from exalting myself!

Concerning this I entreated the Lord **three** times
that it might depart from me.

And He has said to me,

"My **grace** is sufficient for you,
for **power is perfected in weakness."**

Most gladly, therefore, I will rather boast about my weaknesses,
that the **power** of Christ may dwell **in me**.

Therefore, I am well content with weaknesses,
with insults,
with distresses,
with persecutions,
with difficulties,

for Christ's sake; for when I am weak,

then I am strong.

2 Corinthians 12:7-10 NAS

APRIL 5

Jesus called his twelve disciples to him,
and gave them authority to cast out evil spirits
and to heal every kind of sickness and disease. . . .

Jesus sent them out with these instructions: . . .

"Go and announce to them

that the Kingdom of Heaven is near.

Heal the sick,

raise the dead,

cure the lepers,

and cast out demons.

Give as freely as you have received!"

Matthew 10:1, 5,7-8 (TLB). See also Mark 6:7-13, Luke 9:1, 2, 6.

APRIL 6

I called on your name, O LORD,
from the depths of the pit.

You heard my plea:
"Do not close your ears to my cry for relief."

You came near when I called you, and you said,

"Do not fear!"

Lamentations 3:55-57 NIV

Lord, today I am feeling like this . . .

Self-pity is like quicksand,
it will swallow you up.

APRIL 7

ROAD CONSTRUCTION

As we travel, we have experienced many areas of road construction.

The times of growth and change in my personal and spiritual life have been like road constructions.

Heavy traffic causes the road to need repair.

Engineering plans are made,
Financial costs are calculated,
Workers are employed,
Material is ordered,

Work begins.

Machinery is used to tear up the old roadway.
This takes time. What a mess for drivers!

The daily busyness of traffic is slowed down -
Some drivers just take another route.

Traffic is narrowed down to one lane or
rerouted over long detour routes.

New materials are put down over the well prepared foundation.
If good material is not used, rebuilding will have to be done again very soon.

Finally - the new road is ready for traffic again.

Smooth rides again!!!

All growth and change bring **"Road Construction"** to our path, but after its completion the going is smooth again.

APRIL 8

O Lord my God,
I pleaded with You,
and You gave me my health again.

You brought me back from the brink of the grave,
from death itself,
and here I am alive!

Oh, sing to Him you saints of His;
give thanks to His holy name.

His anger lasts a moment;
His favor lasts for life!

Weeping may go on all night, but

in the morning there is JOY!!

Psalm 30:2-5 (TLB)

APRIL 9

L O O K

Into God's Word to find His counsel, direction, and guidance as you walk your walk.

I will bless the Lord who **counsels** me;
He gives me wisdom in the night.
He tells me what to do.

Psalms 16:7 TLB

Blessed Lord, **teach** me Your rules.
I have recited Your laws,
and rejoiced in them more than in riches.

I will meditate upon them and give them my full respect.
I will delight in them and not forget them.

Bless me with life so that I can continue to obey You.

Open my eyes to see wonderful things in Your Word.

I am but a pilgrim here on earth: how I need a map -
and your commands are my chart and guide.
I long for Your instructions more than I can tell.

Psalms 119:12-20 (TLB)

MATILDA A Healing Relationship Bill Adams

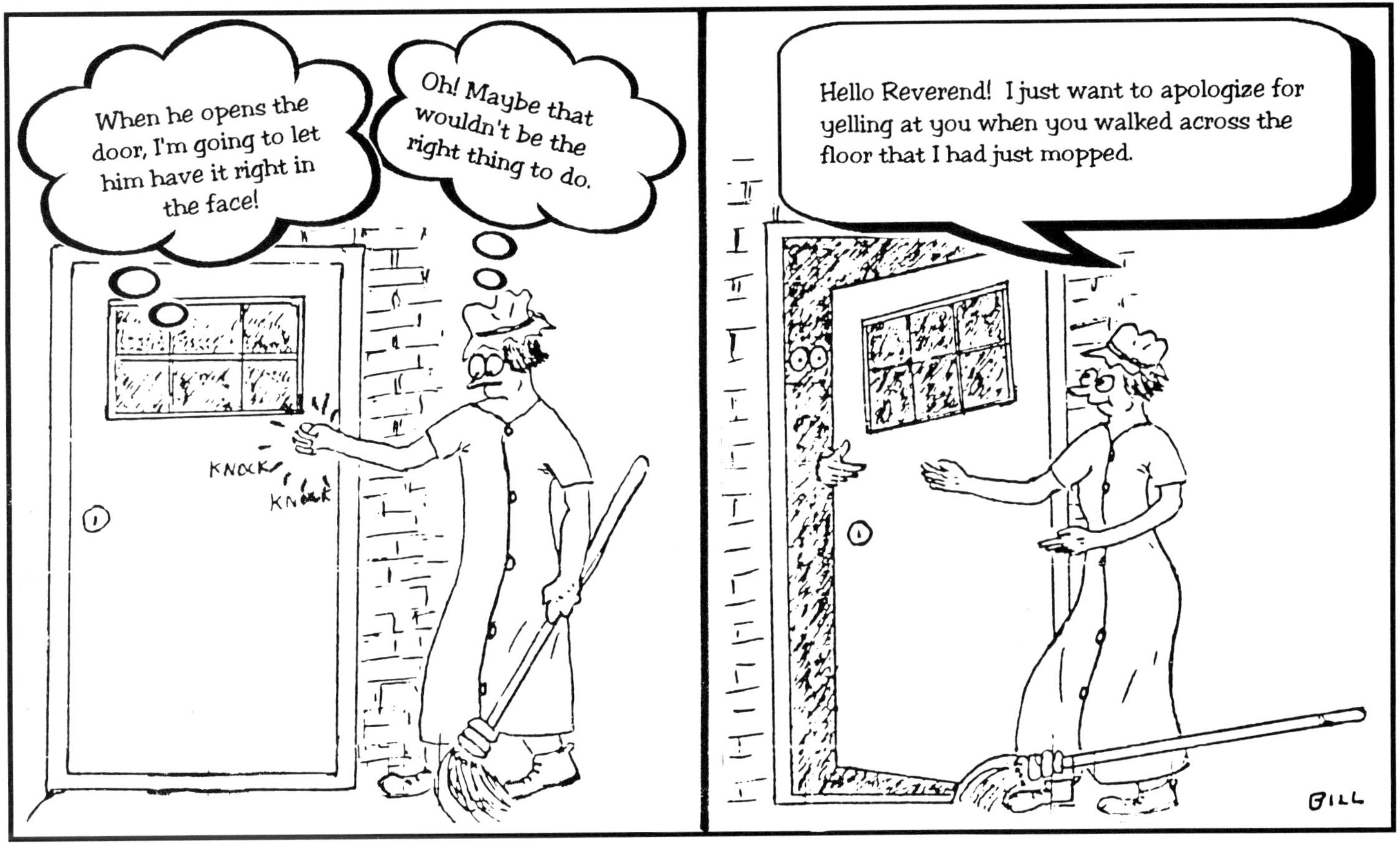
When he opens the door, I'm going to let him have it right in the face!
KNOCK KNOCK
Oh! Maybe that wouldn't be the right thing to do.
Hello Reverend! I just want to apologize for yelling at you when you walked across the floor that I had just mopped.
BILL

APRIL 11

Jesus answered them, . . .

"Behold, an hour is coming,
and has already come,
for you to be scattered,
each to his own home,
and to leave Me alone;
and yet

I am not alone,

because the Father is with me.

These things I have spoken to you,
that in Me you may have ***peace.***

In the world you have tribulation,

but take ***courage;***

I have overcome the world."

John 16:32-33 NAS

APRIL 12

Jesus told them,

> *"Go back to John and tell him about the miracles*
> *you've seen Me do -*
>
> *the blind people I've healed,*
> *the lame people now walking without help,*
> *the cured lepers,*
> *the deaf who hear,*
> *the dead raised to life;*
>
> *and tell him about my preaching the Good News to the poor.*

Then give him this message,

'Blessed are those who don't doubt me.' "

Matthew 11:4-6 (TLB). See also Luke 7:20-22, Isaiah 61:1-2.

APRIL 13

For the eyes of the LORD move to and fro throughout the earth

that He may strongly support those whose heart

is completely His.

2 Chronicles 16:9 NAS

Lord, today I am feeling like this . . .

You may not be responsible for being **down**,
but you are responsible for getting **up**.

APRIL 14

WAITING

Waiting -

For a child to be born . . .
For a child to be placed in our home . . .
For the first smile,
tooth,
steps,
word,
For the first day of school,
report card,
dance recital,
ball game,
and now for the first night this teenager is out without us.
Not knowing is scary, at this late night hour.

The rain gently drips,
the tree frogs sing,
the dog sleeps,
the water flows into the pond and gurgles,
the clock ticks.

Night sounds are magnified in the lonely silence.
Parents wait in fear as a child celebrates her independence.

Lord, fill us with wisdom for the living of these days.

APRIL 15

I **waited patiently** for the LORD;
And He inclined to me, and heard my cry.

He brought me up out of the pit of destruction,
out of the miry clay;
And He set my feet upon a **rock**
making my footsteps firm.

And He put a **new song** in my mouth,
a song of **praise** to our God;
Many will see and fear,
and will trust in the LORD. . . .

I delight to do Thy will, O my God;
Thy Law is within my heart. . . .

Since I am afflicted and needy,
Let the LORD be mindful of me;
Thou art my help and my deliverer;
Do not delay, O my God.

Psalm 40:1-3, 8, 17 NAS

APRIL 16

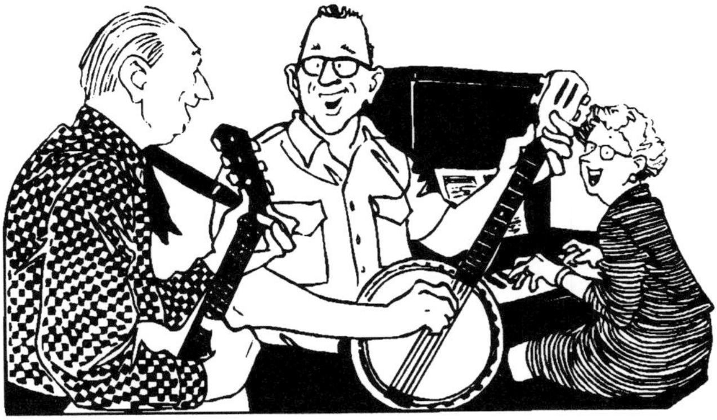

Put on the

GARMENT OF PRAISE

For the spirit of heaviness

Lift up your voice to God

Praise to the Father

And with understanding

O, magnify the LORD

From a spiritual song adapted from Isaiah 61:3

APRIL 17

IT IS WELL WITH MY SOUL

On March 21, 1990, we were in Dayton, Ohio, where Ron was undergoing three hours of neuropsychological testing with a clinical psychologist. To pass the time, I went browsing in a Christian bookstore at the mall.

On the shelf just inside the door was a new book by Timothy Botts. I was so excited to find his new book, *WINDSONGS*! His *DOORPOSTS*, Scripture calligraphic renderings, had blessed and encouraged me so much when I first saw it at Christmas that I ordered myself a copy for my birthday.

WINDSONGS was a book of calligraphic interpretations of hymns and spiritual songs. The pages illustrating the hymn *It Is Well With My Soul* spoke so timely to me of the painful season we were in as we searched for medical answers to Ron's behavioral changes. The book went home with me.

When I shared the book and picture with my bell choir director, she suggested I learn to play a hand bell solo of *It Is Well With My Soul.*

"NO! Not me! I know nothing about music. I am not skilled or confident enough to play a solo!"

She continued to encourage me and even ordered the music for us to begin to practice. She would join me by playing on the harp. I finally agreed to learn the solo as my testimony of God's presence **with** me in this wilderness journey. The performance was scheduled for June 3rd. Later, I realized that this was the date of the surprise retirement party for Ron.

God continued to comfort me and confirm His presence **with** me through this hymn. So many times it would be played on the Christian radio station at just the time I needed to be encouraged by hearing it.

The following January on my birthday, *It Is Well With My Soul* was sung during the worship service at our church in Kansas City. One year after I had played the hand bell solo, the song was sung as a solo at our Kansas City worship service.

God has faithfully and continually encouraged and blessed me by having this hymn played at just the moments I need to hear its message.

The *WINDSONGS* illustration is shared on the May 17-18 page of this *Journal*. The words and music of the hymn are shared on September 17.

APRIL 18

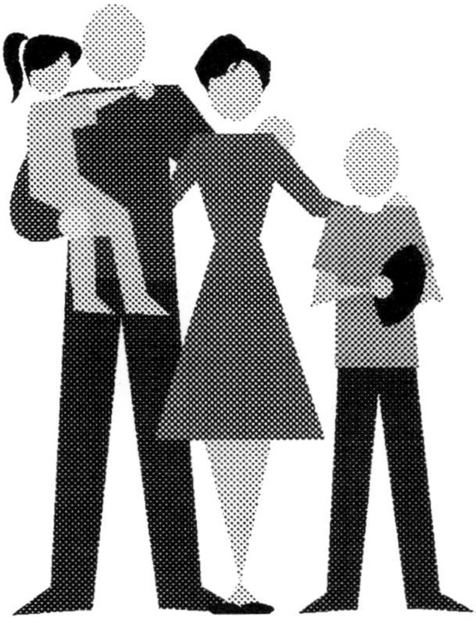

Do you not know that **you** are a **temple of God**,
and that the Spirit of God **dwells in you**?

If any man destroys the **temple of God,**
God will destroy him,
for the **temple of God is holy**
and that is what **you** are.

1 Corinthians 3:16-17 NAS

"**Go** up to the mountains,
bring wood and
rebuild the temple,

(Why?) that I might be pleased with it and be **glorified**,"
says the LORD.

Haggai 1:8 NAS

APRIL 19

Then He went over to the synagogue,
and noticed there a man with a deformed hand.

The Pharisees asked Jesus,

"Is it legal to work by healing on the Sabbath day?"

(They were, of course, hoping He would say "Yes,"
so they could arrest Him!)

This was His answer:

"If you had just one sheep,
and it fell into a well on the Sabbath,
would you work to rescue it that day?
Of course, you would.
And how much more valuable is a person than a sheep!
Yes, it is right to do good on the Sabbath."

Then He said to the man,

"Stretch out your arm."

And as he did, his hand became normal, just like the other one!

Matthew 12:9-13 (TLB). See also Mark 3:1-5, Luke 6:6-10.

APRIL 20

. . . if you have faith as a mustard seed,
you shall say to this mountain,

'Move from here to there,'

and it shall move;
and **nothing** shall be impossible to you.

Matthew 17:20 NAS

Lord, today I am feeling like this . . .

Faith either removes mountains
or tunnels through them.

APRIL 21

EASTER EGG HUNT

A friend has been waiting very long to receive an adopted child.

My son has looked for over two months for housing to meet his growing family's needs. Involvement with them in all their searching, waiting, hopes, and disappointments reminds me of an Easter Egg Hunt.

All over the yard the adults have hidden brightly colored Easter eggs and candy. One special large egg with a **big** prize inside has been hidden in the best hiding place.

The children eagerly **wait** for the signal to **"Go!!"** to **search** for the surprises.

One child rushes and begins grabbing every egg and candy in sight, filling his basket full.

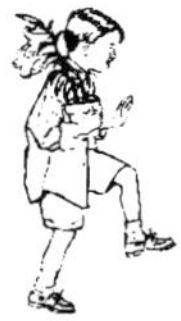

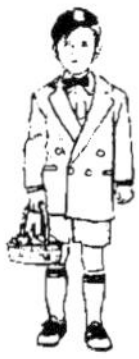

Another child walks slowly around looking for the special prize egg, not touching any other egg.

There's a child who takes the first candy found and stands eating and enjoying the moment.

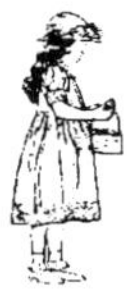

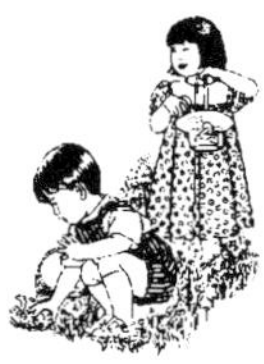

A sister helps her younger brother find and pick up eggs.

Continued on April 22

APRIL 22

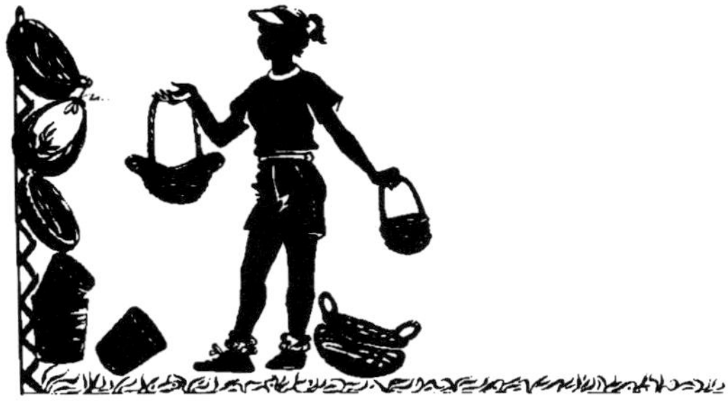

All the time, the parents are shouting instructions and pointing

"Over there!" "Go this way!"
"Look behind that tree" "Hurry!"
"You're close!" "You passed it!"

Wanting their child to find the special **prize** egg -
Wanting the **best** for their child -
Knowing where it is -
But the child has to find it by themselves.

So Close! **open your eyes**

Oops! You missed it.
What you found is good and enjoyable,

But ~ not the very best available.

God's viewpoint of our needs is like an Easter Egg Hunt.

He **knows** what is best for us - what we want and need -
and He plans for us to have it.

But He **waits** for our **obedience** and **effort**
to be at the right place, at the right time,
for us to find His special will for us.

APRIL 23

Even the **wilderness** and **desert** will rejoice in those days;
the desert will blossom with flowers.
Yes, there will be an abundance of flowers and singing and joy!
The deserts will become as green as the Lebanon mountains, as lovely as Mount Carmel's pastures and Sharon's meadows; for the Lord will display his glory there, the excellency of our God.

With this news bring cheer to all **discouraged** ones.

Encourage those who are **afraid.** Tell them,

"**Be strong, fear not**
for your God is coming to destroy your enemies.
He is coming to save you."

and when He comes, **He will**

O p e n the eyes of the blind, and
Unstop the ears of the deaf.
The **lame man will leap** up like a deer, and
those who **could not speak will shout and sing!**

Springs will burst forth in the wilderness,

and streams in the desert.

The parched ground will become a pool,
with springs of water in the thirsty land. . . .

For them all sorrow and all sighing will be gone forever;
only **JOY** and **GLADNESS** will be there.

Isaiah 35:1-7, 10 (TLB)

APRIL 24

The Lord says, "Behold, **I Myself will**

search	for my lost sheep
seek	them out
care	for my sheep
feed	them in good pasture
bind	up the broken
strengthen	the sick

I, Myself will be the **shepherd of My sheep**."

Ezekiel 34:11-16 Paraphrased

So Jesus used this illustration:

"If you had a hundred sheep and one of them strayed away
and was lost in the wilderness,
wouldn't you leave the ninety-nine others to go and
search for the lost one until you found it? . . . "

Luke 15:3-4 (TLB)

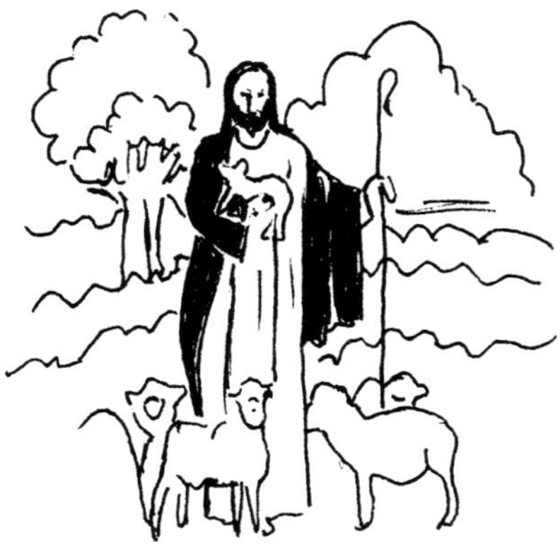

APRIL 25

From: *Windsongs*. By: Timothy Botts (c) 1989.

APRIL 26

For I consider that the **sufferings** of this present time
are not worthy to be compared with the **glory** that
is to be revealed to us.

For the anxious longing of the creation waits
eagerly for the revealing of the sons of God.

For the creation was subjected to futility, not of its own will,
but because of Him who subjected it in **hope**
that the creation itself also will be **set free**
from its slavery to corruption into the freedom
of the **glory** of the children of God.

For we know that the whole creation **groans** and **suffers**
the pains of childbirth together until now.

And not only this, but also we ourselves,
having the first fruits of the Spirit,
even we ourselves groan within ourselves,
waiting eagerly for our adoption as sons,
the redemption of our body.

For in **hope** we have been saved,
but hope that is seen is not hope;
for why does one also hope for what he sees?

But if we hope for what we do not see,
with perseverance we wait eagerly for it.

Romans 8:18-25 NAS

APRIL 27

A woman from Canaan who was living there came to him, pleading,
"Have mercy on me, O Lord, King David's Son!
For my daughter has a demon within her,
and it torments her constantly."

But Jesus gave her no reply - not even a word.

Then His disciples urged Him to send her away.

"Tell her to get going," they said,
"for she is bothering us with all her begging."

Then He said to the woman,

"I was sent to help the Jews -
the lost sheep of Israel - not the Gentiles."

But she came and **worshiped** him and pled again,

"Sir, help me!"

"It doesn't seem right to take bread from the children
and throw it to the dogs," He said.

"Yes, it is!" she replied,
"For even the puppies beneath the table are permitted to eat the crumbs that fall."

"Woman," Jesus told her,
"your faith is large, and your request is granted."

And her daughter was healed right then.

Matthew 15:22-28 (TLB). See also Mark 7:25-30.

APRIL 28

Count to ten when you are upset

OUR
FATHER
WHO
ART
IN
HEAVEN
HALLOWED
BE
THY
NAME

Lord, today I am feeling like this . . .

APRIL 29

RAIN AND RAINBOWS

Rain, Rain, Rain
Days of Rain
Life is controlled by the rain.

It confines us to indoor activities
We run to the warmth and protection of shelter places.

Some days are violent days as the thunder and lightning
and hail roll across the skies.

All activities cease, as the violence forces us to seek protection.

then

After days of rain -

Just when we think we can't stand any more rain
The sun comes out

unexpectedly

and there in the eastern sky is a rainbow -

a double rainbow!!

bright, crisp, clear colors of the complete inner rainbow;
misty, blended colors of the complete outer rainbow.

We are frozen in awe,
absorbing the wonder and miracle of this gift

a double rainbow!!

Continued on April 30

APRIL 30

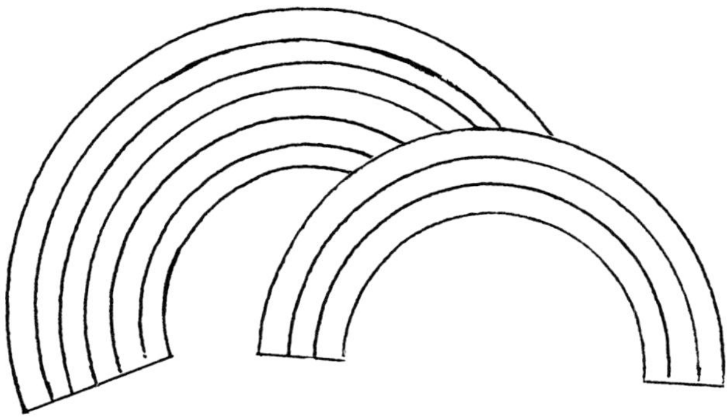

We don't run for shelter now.
We stand absorbing this brief moment
in the wonder of creation.
Realizing that after the storms
A message of hope has come.

God is saying,

"Never again will floods overtake you:
I am **with** you through the storms of life."

No longer is it necessary to seek protection to hide from the storm
Color and Joy and Freedom have returned to life.

Go in the **joy** of the **rainbow**
To share in the freedom of renewed life.

"I set My bow in the cloud, and it shall be for a sign of a covenant between Me and the earth." Genesis 9:13 NAS

Written April 29, 1989

MAY 1

So the people **grumbled** at Moses, saying,

"What shall we drink?"

Then he cried out to the LORD,
and the LORD showed him a tree;
and he threw it into the waters,
and the water became sweet.

There He made for them a statute and regulation,
and there He tested them.

And He said,

"**If you will give earnest heed to the voice** of the LORD your God,

and **do** what is right in His sight,

and **give** ear to His commandments,

and **keep** all His statues,

I will put none of the diseases on you which I have put on the Egyptians; for

I, the LORD, am your HEALER."

Then they came to Elim
where there were **twelve springs of water** and **seventy date palms**,

and they **camped** there beside the **waters**.

Exodus 15:24-27 NAS

MAY 2

And not only this,

but we also **exult in our tribulations**,

knowing that

tribulation brings about perseverance

and perseverance proven character

and proven character hope

and hope does not disappoint,

because

the LOVE of God has been P
O
U
R
E
D OUT

within our hearts through the Holy Spirit
who was given to us.

For while we were still helpless,

at the right time

Christ died for the ungodly.

Romans 5:3-5 NAS

MAY 3

"Think back over the journey you made," he replied, "and tell me what lessons you learned on the way."

She was silent for a while as she reviewed the whole journey, which had seemed so terribly long and in some places so cruelly difficult and even impossible. She thought of the altars which she had built along the way; of the time when she had stood with him at the trysting-place in the Valley, when he had called her to follow him to the heights. She remembered the walk to the foot of the mountains; the first meeting with Suffering and Sorrow and of learning to accept their help; she recalled the shock of what had seemed such a heartbreaking detour down into the desert, and of the things which she had seen there.

Then their journey along the shores of Loneliness; the empty cove which the sea had filled to the brim; and then the agony of disappointment and frustration experienced in the wilderness when the path once again had turned away from the High Places. She remembered crossing the great sea-wall, walking through the woods and valleys until the rapturous moment when the path had turned back toward the mountains. Her thoughts turned to the Precipice of Injury, the Forests of Danger and Tribulation, the great storm during which they had sheltered in the hut. And then the mist - the endless mist, and the awful moment when the path suddenly led down into the Valley of Loss, and the nightmare abyss of horror into which she had looked when she had thought of turning back.

She recalled the descent down into the Valley of Loss and the peace she had found there before reascending to the heights in the aerial chairs, and of the days spent in that place where she had been prepared for her burial. Then that last agonizing ascent, and the cave where they sheltered from the floods and where she had been tempted to cast away the promises. Then the spring called Marah, and finally the mist-shrouded grave up among the peaks where she had been bound to the altar. How little she had imagined, when first she set out on that strange journey, what lay ahead of her and the things which she would be called upon to pass through. So for a long time she sat silent - remembering, wondering, and thankful.

Continued on May 4

MAY 4

At last she put her hand in his and said softly, "My Lord, I will tell you what I learned."

"Tell me," he answered gently.

"First," said she, "I learned that I must accept with joy all that you allowed to happen to me on the way and everything to which the path led me! That I was never to try to evade it but to accept it and lay down my own will on the altar and say, 'Behold me, I am thy little handmaiden Acceptance-with-Joy.' "

He nodded without speaking, and she went on, "Then I learned that I must bear all that others were allowed to do against me and to forgive with no trace of bitterness and to say to thee, 'Behold me - I am thy little handmaiden Bearing-with-Love,' that I may receive power to bring good out of this evil."

Again he nodded, and she smiled still more sweetly and happily.

The third thing that I learned was that you, my Lord, never regarded me as I actually was, lame and weak and crooked and cowardly. You saw me as I would be when you had done what you promised and had brought me to the High Places, when it could be truly said, 'There is none that walks with such a queenly ease, nor with such grace, as she.' You always treated me with the same love and graciousness as though I were a queen already and not wretched little Much-Afraid." Then she looked up into his face and for a little time could say no more, but at last she added, "My Lord, I cannot tell you how greatly I want to regard others in the same way."

A very lovely smile broke out on his face at that, but he still said nothing, only nodded for the third time and waited for her to continue.

"The fourth thing," said she with a radiant face, "Was really the first I learned up here. Every circumstance in life, no matter how crooked and distorted and ugly it appears to be, if it is reacted to in love and forgiveness and obedience to your will can be transformed."

Continued on May 5

MAY 5

"Therefore I begin to think, my Lord, you purposely allow us to be brought into contact with the bad and evil things that you want changed. Perhaps that is the very reason why we are here in this world, where sin and sorrow and suffering and evil abound, so that we may let you teach us so to react to them, that out of them we can create lovely qualities to live forever. That is the only really satisfactory way of dealing with evil, not simply binding it so that it cannot work harm, but whenever possible overcoming it with good."

At last he spoke, "You have learned well, Grace and Glory. Now I will add one thing more. It was these lessons which you have learned which enabled me to change you from limping, crippled Much-Afraid into Grace and Glory with the hinds' feet. Now you are able to run, leaping on the mountains and able to follow me wherever I go, so that we need never be parted again.

"So remember this; as long as you are willing to be Acceptance-with-Joy and Bearing-in-Love, you can never again become crippled, and you will be able to go wherever I lead you. You will be able to go down into the Valley of the world to work with me there, for that is where the evil and sorrowful and ugly things are which need to be overcome.

"Accept and bear and obey the Law of Love, and nothing will be able to cripple your hinds' feet or to separate you from me. This is the secret of the High Places, Grace and Glory, it is the lovely and perfect law of the whole universe. It is this that makes the radiant joy of the Heavenly Places." Then he rose to his feet, drew her up beside him, and said, "Now use your hinds' feet again, for I am going to lead you to another part of the mountain."

Hinds' Feet on High Places, Hannah Hurnard, pages 239-243

MAY 6

No longer do I call you slaves,
for the slave does not know what his master is doing;
but **I have called you friends,**
for all things that I have heard from My Father
I have made known to you.

John 15:15 NAS

Lord, today I am feeling like this . . .

A **friend** is someone who walks in,
when the rest of the world walks out.

MAY 7

To my child,

May you receive these words as your mother speaking to your soul.

I am writing this to ask your forgiveness.

For nine months I carried you close to my heart and loved you from the beginning. God formed you and did weave you in my womb. You were fearfully and wonderfully made. Jesus has always lived in you from conception.

My pain in the delivery was soon forgotten in the joy of seeing you. You were beautiful! And I loved you!!

But as the demands of life and the reality of child rearing began to consume me, I found that I was not prepared for the job of loving you the way God planned for mothers to love their children. I had my own hurts from my parents to work through, and hurts from other relationships. And I raised you the same way I had been raised. It was all I knew.

When I hurt you by my actions or words, it came from my own hurts. Please forgive me.

When I said things that you received as rejection or shame or condemnation, please forgive me.

When I forgot to do things for you, please forgive me.

When I wasn't there for you, please forgive me.

In my own way, I loved you very deeply and I still do. And now my heart cries out to have the opportunity to love you again as a baby. I long to take you in my arms and hold you and love on you and let you nurse from the good milk of the Word of God. I want you to take your time nursing and get your fill of God's love that He speaks to you in His Word.

When you are full of the milk of God's Word and His Love, please forgive me as Jesus did the woman at the well. He knew all the hurtful things she had done, and He forgave her with God's love. Please forgive me.

I love you with God's love, grace, and mercy.

Written June, 1991

MAY 8

BUT AS FOR ME

But if serving the LORD seems undesirable to you,
then choose for yourselves this day whom you will serve . . .
But as for me and my household,
we will serve the LORD.

Joshua 24:15 NIV

But as for me,
by Thine abundant lovingkindness I will enter Thy house,
at Thy holy temple I will bow in reverence for Thee.

Psalm 5:7 NAS

But as for me,
I shall walk in my integrity;
redeem me, and be gracious to me.
My foot stands on a level place;
in the congregations I shall bless the LORD.

Psalm 26:11,12 NAS

But as for me,
when they were sick, my clothing was sackcloth;
I humbled my soul with fasting;
and my prayer kept returning to my bosom.

Psalm 35:13 NAS

But as for me,
I am like a green olive tree in the house of God;
I trust in the lovingkindness of God forever and ever.
I will give Thee thanks forever, because Thou hast done it,
and I will wait on Thy name, for it is good,
in the presence of Thy godly ones.

Psalm 52:8,9 NAS

MAY 9

Which BODY will you choose?

Seven things the Lord hates Proverbs 6:16-19

Proud look
False witness that breathes out lies
Lying tongue
Heart that devises wicked schemes
One who sows discord among brothers
Hands that shed innocent blood
Feet quick to run to evil

Child-ish **Pride is the root of problems**

Old Body - Selfish

When I was a child, I used to speak as a child, think as a child, reason as a child. . . .

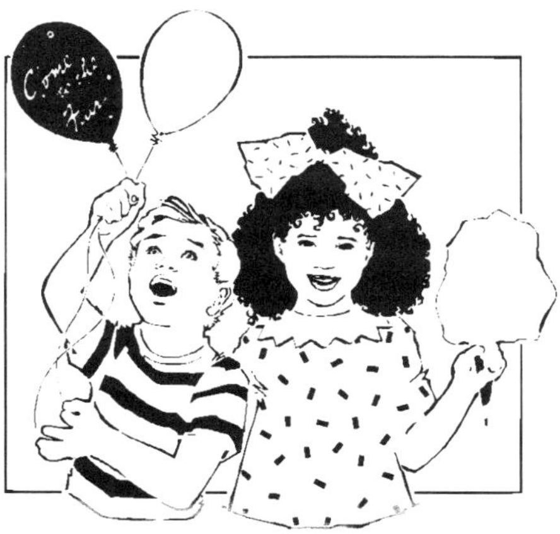

Continued on May 10

MAY 10

Which BODY will you choose?

Seven pieces of armor Ephesians 6:11-18

Helmet of salvation
Breastplate of righteousness
Belt of truth
Shield of faith
Shoes of gospel of peace
Sword of Word of God
Prayer at all times in the Spirit

Child-like **Humble**
New Body - Love

When I became an adult, I did away with childish things.
1 Corinthians 13:11 NAS

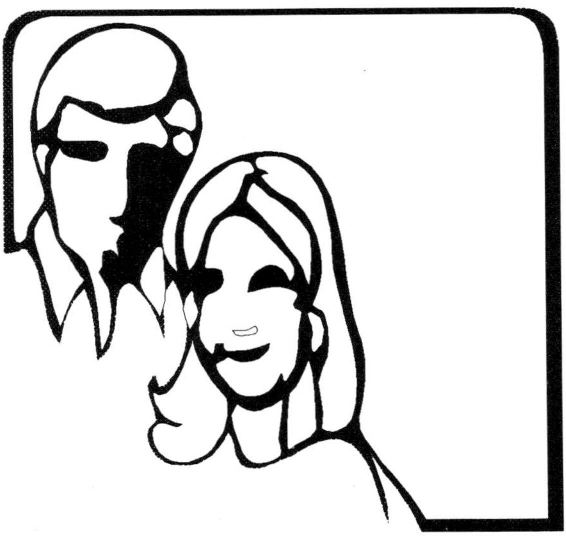

MAY 11

So John was beheaded in the prison,
and his head was brought on a tray and given to the girl,
who took it to her mother.

Then John's disciples came for his body and buried it,
and came to tell Jesus what had happened.

As soon as Jesus heard the news,
He went off by himself
in a boat
to a remote area
to be alone.

But the crowds saw where He was headed,
and followed by land from many villages.

So when Jesus came out of the wilderness,
a vast crowd was waiting for Him and

He pitied them and healed their sick.

Matthew 14:10-14 (TLB)

Jesus, I am consumed with my grief. I invite You to go **with** me on this wilderness journey. I want to be alone with you. Knowing that You, too, grieved gives me comfort. Help me to see others' pain in the midst of my own.

MAY 12

O LORD, be gracious to us;
we have **waited** for Thee.
Be Thou their **strength every morning**,
our salvation also in the **time of distress**. . . .

Who among us can live with the **consuming fire**?
Who among us can live with **continual burning**?

He who **walks righteously**, and
speaks with sincerity,
he who **rejects** unjust gain, and
shakes his hands so that they hold **no bribe**;
he who **stops** his ears from hearing about bloodshed,
and **shuts** his eyes from looking upon evil;

He will dwell on the **heights;**
His refuge will be the impregnable **rock**;
His **bread** will be given him;
His **water** will be sure.

Isaiah 33:2, 14-16 NAS

MAY 13

And in the same way the Spirit also helps our weakness;

for **we do not know how to pray as we should**,

but the Spirit Himself intercedes for us
with groanings too deep for words;

and He who searches the hearts
knows what the mind of the Spirit is,
because He intercedes for the saints
according to the **will of God**.

And we **know** that God causes **all things**
to work together for **good**
to those who **love God,**
to those who are called
according to His Purpose.

Romans 8:26-28 NAS

MAY 14

come HOLY SPIRIT come

P

O

U

R

Your healing **oil of love**

into ______________ and meet __________ at ___________ point of need.

List your needs that you want the Holy Spirit to meet for you.

1.____

2.____

3. ____

4. ____

5. ____

MAY 15

Eight months before Ron's death, I was at a retreat with the women from our church. During a worship time, a prophetic word was spoken to the whole group:

"God wants to put a new garment on you."

Immediately, I knew that I had to become like an infant and raise my arms to the Heavenly Father for Him to put a new garment on me. At that moment I **knew** that the garment for me was widowhood. And in my emotions I had to raise my arms to have that garment put on.

As I did so, flashbacks to dreams God had given me and the truth of their meanings reassured me that the ultimate healing is death and eternal life. I had feelings of guilt and inadequacy, but after I asked two friends to pray with me, the burden was lifted.

Even though I cried a long time as the truth sank in, it was a cleansing crying that washed away my denial of the truth of Ron's illness.

And God's peace and joy returned from the knowledge that He cared so much for Ron and I that He visited me with this revelation and sent friends to support me in prayer.

. . . the mantle (garment) of **praise** instead of a spirit of fainting. . . .
For He has clothed me with garments of **salvation**,
He has wrapped me with a **robe of righteousness**. . . .

Isaiah 61:3,10 NAS

MAY 16

They landed at Gennesaret.

The news of their arrival spread quickly throughout the city,
and soon people were rushing around,

telling everyone to bring in their sick to be healed.

The sick begged Him to let them touch even the tassel of His robe,

and all who did were **healed**.

Matthew 14:34-36 (TLB). See also Mark 6:53-56.

MAY 17

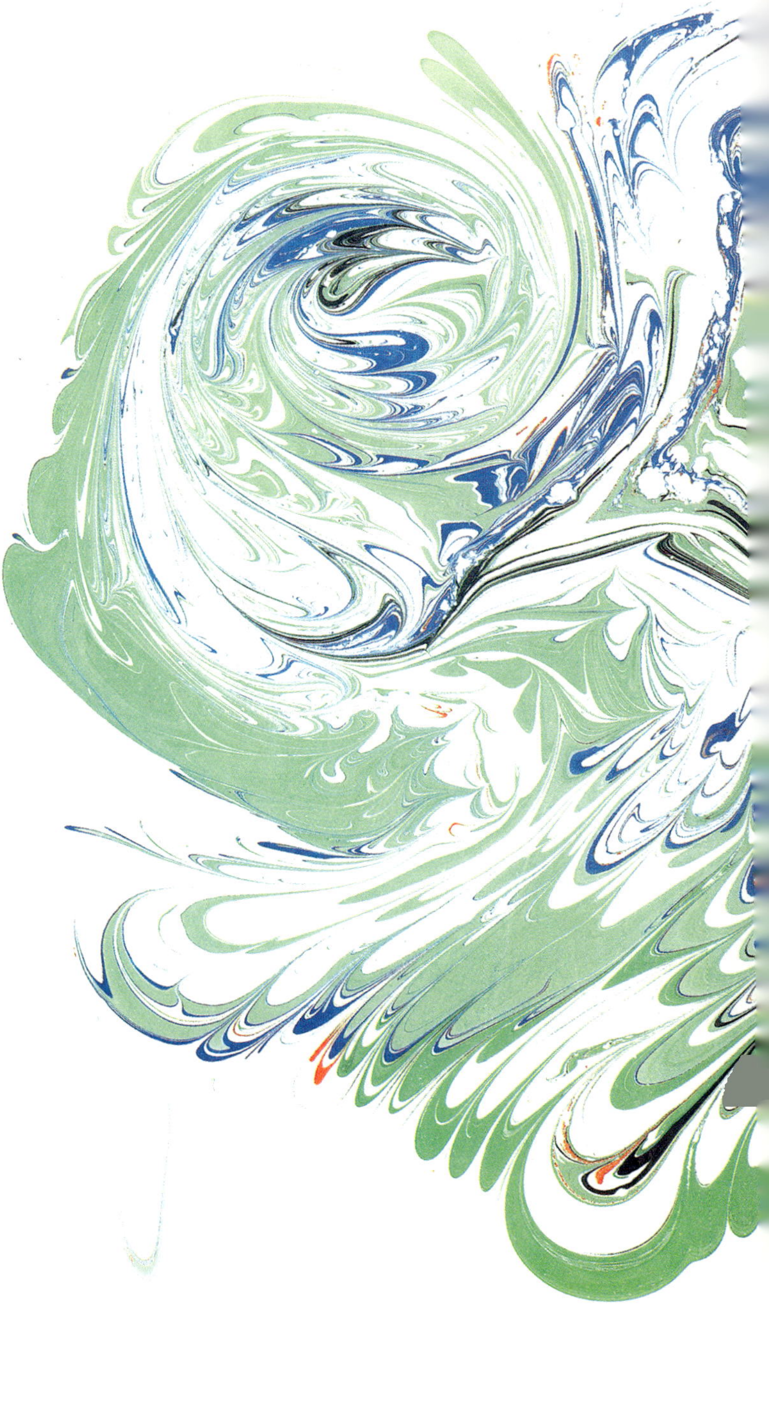

MAY 18

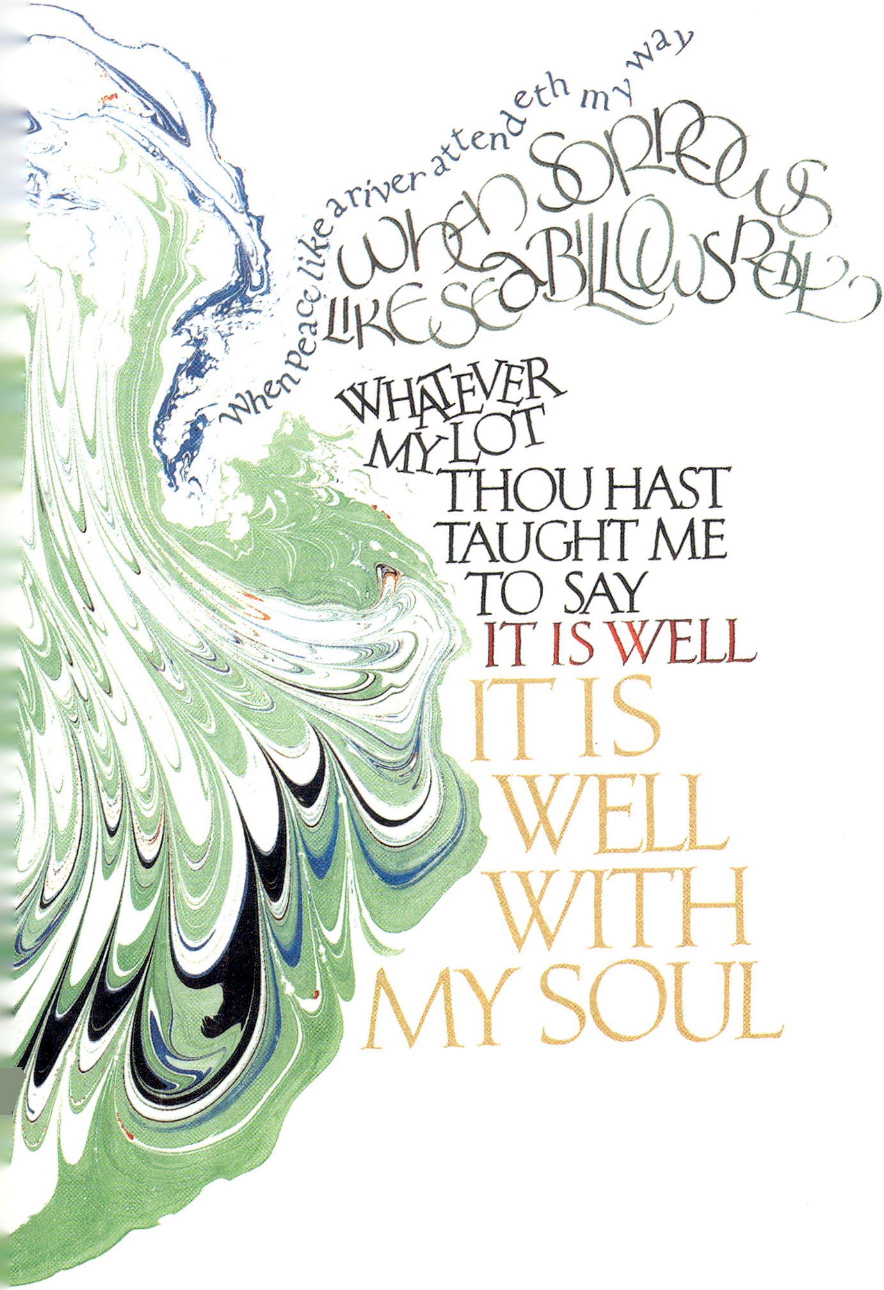
When peace like a river attendeth my way
WHEN SORROWS
LIKE SEA BILLOWS ROLL
WHATEVER
MY LOT
THOU HAST
TAUGHT ME
TO SAY
IT IS WELL
IT IS
WELL
WITH
MY SOUL

From: *Windsongs.* By: Timothy Botts (c) 1989.
Used by permission of Tyndale House Publishers, Inc.

MAY 19

Remember my affliction and my wandering,
the wormwood and bitterness.
Surely my soul remembers
And is bowed down within me.

This I recall to my mind,
Therefore I have **hope**.

The LORD'S **lovingkindnesses** indeed never cease,
For His **compassions** never fail.
They are new **every** morning;

Great is thy faithfulness.

"The LORD is My portion," says my soul,
"Therefore I have **hope** in Him."

The LORD is **good** to those who **wait** for Him,
To the person who **seeks** Him.

It is good that he **waits silently**
For the **salvation** of the LORD.

Lamentations 3:19-26 NAS

MAY 20

For we know that if the earthly tent which is our house is torn down,
we have a building from God,
a house not made with hands,
eternal in the heavens.

For indeed in this house we groan,
longing to be clothed with our dwelling from heaven;
inasmuch as we, having put it on,
shall not be found naked.

For indeed while we are in this tent,
we groan, being burdened,
because we do not want to be unclothed,
but to be clothed,
in order that what is mortal may be swallowed up by life.

Now He who prepared us for this very purpose is God,
who gave to us the Spirit as a pledge.

Therefore, being always of **good courage,**
and knowing that while we are at home in the body
we are absent from the Lord -

for we walk by faith, not by sight -

we are of good courage, I say,
and prefer rather to be absent from the body
and to be at home with the Lord.

Therefore also we have as our ambition,
whether at home or absent,
to be pleasing to Him.

2 Corinthians 5:1-9 NAS

MAY 21

Set your mind on the things above,

not on the things that are on earth.

Colossians 3:2 NAS

Lord, today I am feeling like this . . .

Your mind - like a parachute
has to be O P E N to work.

MAY 22

At the Wednesday prayer ministry, I asked for prayer for my hurting back. A new girl, who did not know my circumstances, began praying and then she said,

> "You are carrying a heavy burden."

The following Monday, as I played golf with Ron, I realized that my golf bag was very heavy on my shoulder. I decided to take out three clubs I seldom used. The Lord spoke to me saying,

> "Lighten your burden."

So I planned to lighten the golf bag by removing three clubs.
The Lord spoke again,

> "Lighten your burden."

I then knew God wanted me to lighten the emotional burden I had been carrying. I had to give up the following three burdens about Ron's illness:

1. Guilt: I did not cause the illness
2. False expectations: I cannot heal it by prayer, preparing certain foods, or finding the "right" doctor
3. Fear of the future

Name three "clubs" you can eliminate that will lighten the burden on your back.

1.____

2.____

3.____

For My yoke is easy and My burden is light. Matthew 11:28-30 NIV

MAY 23

"But for you who revere my name,
the sun of righteousness will rise with healing in its wings.

And you will go out and leap like calves released from the stall.

Then you will trample down the wicked;
they will be ashes under the soles of your feet
on the day when I do these things,"
says the LORD Almighty.

Malachi 4:2-3 NIV

MAY 24

Then a demon-possessed man
he was both blind and unable to talk

was brought to Jesus, and

Jesus healed him

so that he could both speak and see.

The crowd was amazed.

"Maybe Jesus is the Messiah!" they exclaimed.

Matthew 12:22 (TLB). See also Luke 11:14-15.

MAY 25

In the year of King Uzziah's **death,**
I **saw** the Lord sitting on a throne,
lofty and exalted,
with the train of His robe
filling the temple.

Seraphim stood above Him,
each having six wings;
with two he covered his face, and
with two he covered his feet, and
with two he flew.

And one called out to another and said,

"Holy, Holy, Holy
is the LORD of hosts,
The whole earth is full of His glory."

Isaiah 6:1-3 NAS

Lord, at the point of death, may I be able to **worship** You
in all Your Holiness, as Isaiah did.

MAY 26

. . . greater is He who is **in you**

than he who is in the world.

1 John 4:4 NAS

Lord, today I am feeling like this . . .

When someone's Bible falls apart,
you can be sure that they are all together.

MAY 27

For this reason, I bow my knees before the Father,
from whom every family in heaven and on earth derives its name,
that He would grant you, according to the riches of His glory,
to be strengthened with power through His Spirit in the inner man;
so that Christ may dwell in your hearts through faith;
and that you, being rooted and grounded in love,
may be able to comprehend with all the saints
what is the breadth and length and height and depth,
and to know the love of Christ which surpasses knowledge,
that you may be filled up to all the fulness of God.

Ephesians 3:14-19 NAS

As you therefore have received Christ Jesus the Lord,
so walk in Him,
having been firmly rooted
and now being built up in Him
and established in your faith,
just as you were instructed,
and overflowing with gratitude.

Colossians 2:6,7 NAS

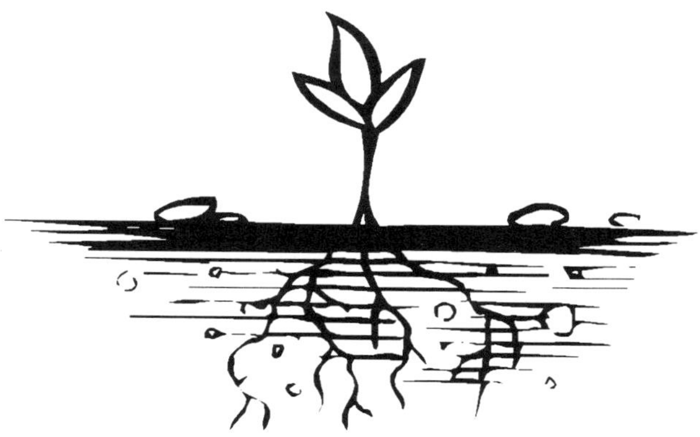

MAY 28

Around my house are shrubs planted among small white stones. Before the stones were put down, thick plastic was laid down. That plastic is tearing and the weeds are beginning to come up.

How do I deal with the weeds?

1. Put chemical weed killer on them.

2. Continually pull each one out by hand.

3. Go over them with a weed eater.

4. Take all the rocks out. Clean the area. Lay new plastic. Put back the stones and add new stones.

In my role as Caregiver, searching for medical answers for the disease, learning to cope with limitations, learning to make daily decisions . . .

How do I handle this?

1. Search for medicine to cure or cover up pain.

2. Keep searching for a new doctor or treatment.

3. Ignore or take lightly the symptoms.

4. Ask for God's wisdom and guidance to get to the root of the problem. Then do all hard work to bring either healing or acceptance and comfort.

Look after each other so that not one of you will fail to find God's best blessings.

Watch out that no bitterness takes root among you, for as it springs up it causes deep trouble, hurting many in their spiritual lives.
Hebrews 12:15 (TLB)

MAY 29

For we who live are constantly being delivered over to death for Jesus' sake, that the life of Jesus also may be manifested in our mortal flesh.

So death works in us, but life in you.

But having the same spirit of faith . . .
we also **believe**,
therefore also we speak;
knowing that He who raised the Lord Jesus will raise us also with Jesus and will present us with you.

For all things are for your sakes,
that the grace which is spreading to more and more people
may cause the giving of thanks to abound to the glory of God.

Therefore, **we do not lose heart,**

but though our outer man is decaying,
yet our inner man is being **renewed** day by day.

For momentary, light affliction is producing for us
an eternal weight of glory far beyond all comparison,
while we look not at the things which are seen,
but at the things which are not seen;
for the things which are seen are temporal,
but the things which are not seen are eternal.

2 Corinthians 4:11-18 NAS

MAY 30

When I started to play the hand bells at church, I knew nothing about music or bell playing, except that I loved to hear them played and I wanted to learn to play. The bell choir director was a patient teacher. She even marked my music by the note names and right or left hand. I began to realize my own personal growth and the spiritual lessons I have gained by learning to play the bells. When we played *Praise and Alleluia* I realized that is why I play bells. To say **"praise and alleluia!!"** to God for all the new music He has brought into and played in my life.

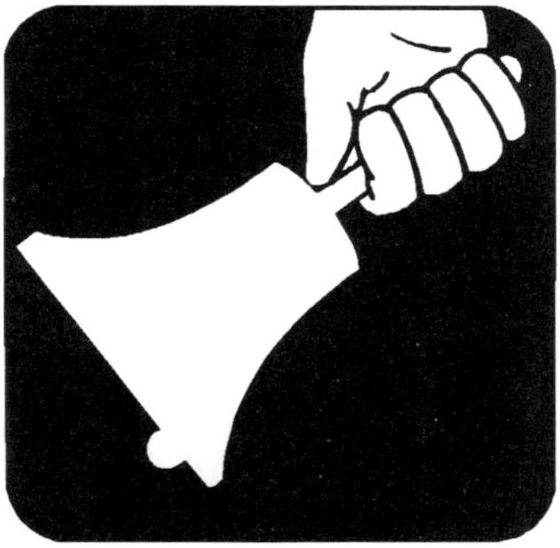

Hold tight to the handle
    Look for and pick up the correct bell
        Wrong note rung cannot be brought back,
        just keep on playing the next measures
            Keep my eyes on the Director
The Director can hear the total music
    Players can hear themselves and those close to them
        Learn the notes, follow the notes written by experts
            Wait my turn to play my note
Sometimes I play a lot and sometimes not very often
    Ask for help from my neighbor when I have
    too many bells to play at one time
        I play only my notes, not someone else's notes
            Look ahead . . .

MAY 31

PEDAL

At first I saw God as my observer, my judge, keeping track of the things I did wrong, so as to know whether I merited heaven or hell when I die. He was out there, sort of like the president. I recognized His picture when I saw it, but I didn't really **know** Him.

But later on when I learned to know Him personally, it seemed as though life was rather like a bike ride, but it was a tandem bike, and I noticed that God was in the back helping me pedal.

I don't know just when it was that He suggested we change places, but life has not been the same since, life with God, that is. God makes life exciting!

When I had control, I knew the way. It was rather boring but predictable. It was the shortest distance between two points.

But when He took the lead, He knew delightful long cuts, up mountains, and through rocky places and at breakneck speeds; it was all I could do to hang on!!!! Even though it looked like madness, He said, **"Pedal!"**

I worried and was anxious and asked, "Where are you taking me?" He laughed and didn't answer, and I started to **trust.**

I forgot my boring life and entered into the adventure. And when I'd say "I'm scared," He'd lean back and touch my hand.

Continued on the next page

MAY 31

He took me to people with gifts that I needed, gifts of healing, acceptance and joy. They gave me their gifts to take on my journey, our journey, God's and mine.

And we were off again. He said. "Give the gifts away; they're extra baggage, too much weight." So I did, to the people we met, and I found that in giving I received, and still our burden was light.

I did not trust Him at first, in control of my life. I thought He'd wreck it, but He knows bike secrets, knows how to make it bend to take sharp corners, jump to clear high rocks, fly to shorten scary passages.

And I am learning to shut up and pedal in the strangest places, and I'm beginning to enjoy the view and the cool breeze on my face with my delightful constant companion, God.

And when I'm sure I just can't do any more, He just smiles and says . . .

. . . "PEDAL" . . .

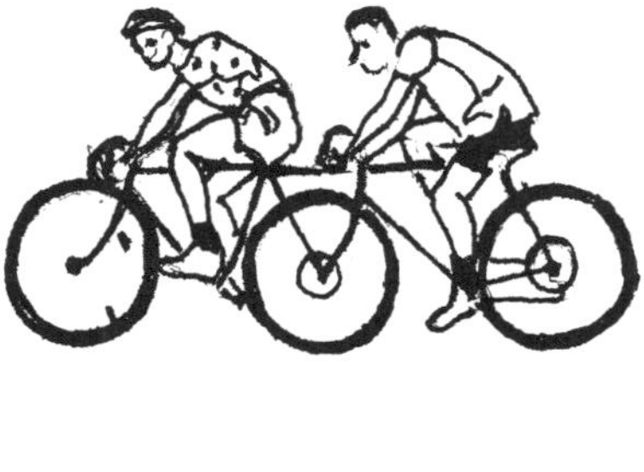

Author Unkown

JUNE 1

Do you remember Mary, who poured the costly perfume on Jesus' feet and wiped them with her hair? Well, her brother Lazarus, who lived in Bethany with Mary and her sister Martha, was sick. So the two sisters sent a message to Jesus telling Him, "Sir, **your good friend is very, very sick**."

But when Jesus heard about it He said, *"The purpose of his illness is not death, but for the glory of God. I, the Son of God, will receive glory from this situation."*

Although Jesus was very fond of Martha, Mary, and Lazarus, He stayed where He as for the next two days and made no move to go to them. Finally, after two days, He said to His disciples, *"Let's go to Judea."*

But His disciples objected. "Master," they said, "only a few days ago the Jewish leaders in Judea were trying to kill you. Are you going there again?"

Jesus replied. *"There are twelve hours of daylight every day, and during every hour of it a man can walk safely and not stumble. Only at night is there danger of a wrong step, because of the dark."* Then He said, *"Our friend Lazarus has gone to sleep, but now I will go and waken him!"*

The disciples, thinking Jesus meant Lazarus was having a good night's rest, said. "That means he is getting better!" But Jesus meant Lazarus had died.

Then He told them plainly, *"Lazarus is dead. And for your sake I am glad I wasn't there, for this will give you another opportunity to believe in me. Come, let's go to him."*

Thomas, nicknamed "The Twin" said to his fellow disciples, "Let's go too - and die with him."

When they arrived at Bethany, they were told that Lazarus had already been in his tomb for four days. Bethany was only a couple of miles down the road from Jerusalem, and many of the Jewish leaders had come to pay their respects and to console Martha and Mary on their loss. When Martha got word that Jesus was coming, she went to meet him. But Mary stayed at home.

Martha said to Jesus, "Sir, if You had been here, my brother wouldn't have died. And even now it's not too late, for I know that God will bring my brother back to life again, if you will only ask Him to."

Jesus told her, *"Your brother will come back to life again."*

"Yes," Martha said, "when everyone else does, on Resurrection Day."

Jesus told her, *"I am the one who raises the dead and gives them life again. Anyone who believes in Me, even though he dies like anyone else, shall live again. He is given eternal life for believing in Me and shall never perish. Do you believe this, Martha?"*

Continued on June 2

JUNE 2

"Yes, Master," she told Him. "I believe You are the Messiah, the Son of God, the one we have so long awaited."

Then she left Him and returned to Mary and calling her aside from the mourners, told her, "He is here and wants to see you." So Mary went to Him at once.

Now Jesus had stayed outside the village, at the place where Martha met Him. When the Jewish leaders who were at the house trying to console Mary saw her leave so hastily, they assumed she was going to Lazarus's tomb to weep; so they followed her.

When Mary arrived where Jesus was, she fell down at His feet, saying "Sir, IF You had been here my brother would still be alive."

When Jesus saw her weeping and the Jewish leaders wailing with her, He was moved with indignation and deeply troubled. *"Where is He buried?"* He asked them. They told Him, "Come and See."

Tears came to Jesus' eyes.

"They were close friends," the Jewish leaders said. "See how much He loved him."

But some said, "This fellow healed a blind man - why couldn't He keep Lazarus from dying?" And again Jesus was moved with deep anger. Then they came to the tomb. It was a cave with a heavy stone rolled across its door.

"Roll the stone aside," Jesus told them.

But Martha, the dead man's sister, said, "By now the smell will be terrible, for he has been dead four days."

"But didn't I tell you that you will see a wonderful miracle from God if you believe?" Jesus asked her.

So they rolled the stone aside. Then Jesus looked up to heaven and said, *"Father, thank you for hearing me. (You always hear Me, of course, but I said it because of all these people standing here, so that they will believe you sent Me.)*

Then He SHOUTED, *"LAZARUS, COME OUT!"*

And Lazarus came - bound up in the grave cloth, his face muffled in a head swath.

Jesus told them, *"Unwrap him and let him go!"*

And so at last many of the Jewish leaders who were with Mary and saw it happen, finally believed on Him.

John 11:1-45 (TLB)

JUNE 3

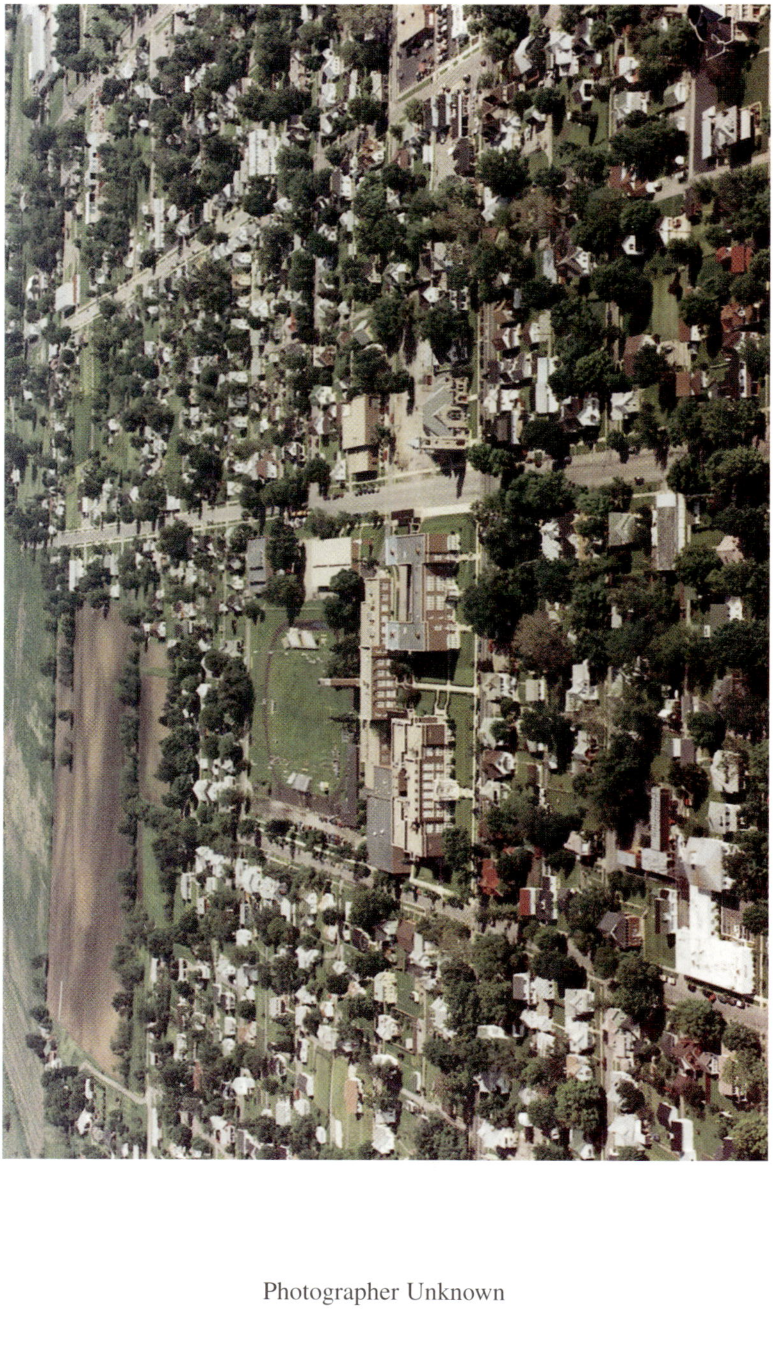

Photographer Unknown

JUNE 4

GOD'S VIEWPOINT

At Ron's retirement party on June 3, 1990, he was given an aerial photograph of the McClain High School campus in Greenfield, Ohio, where he had been a coach and the athletic director for eighteen years. The photographer also gave us the other viewpoints of the campus and the town that he had taken.

One picture of the whole town really spoke to me. It showed how God looks down on earth and sees everything in perspective. We tend to get caught up in our own little area.

God **sees** everyone from **His viewpoint.**

At the last bell choir gathering before I left Greenfield, we played simply for the joy of playing together. The director gave me a tape of all the selections we had performed publicly in the past. It was the first time I had heard the music from the listener's viewpoint.

This time I **heard** from **God's viewpoint.**

When I had played the handbells, I was so intent on just the bells I was responsible for and my music that I never really heard the blending and harmony of the total sound.

These two events **O P E N E D** me to
seeing and hearing anew from **God's viewpoint.**

For His eyes are upon the ways of a man,
And He sees all his steps.

Job 34:21 NAS

JUNE 5

He will turn the hearts of the fathers to their children,

and the hearts of the children to their fathers. . . .

Malachi 4:6 NIV

JUNE 6

Enemies lock us inside	Now Jericho was tightly shut because of the sons of Israel; no one went out and no one came in.
God's in Control	And the LORD said to Joshua, "See, I have given Jericho into your hand, with its king and the valiant warriors. You shall march around the city, all the
Test faith	men of war circling the city once. You shall do so for six days. Also seven priests shall carry seven trumpets . . .
Follow command details	then on the seventh day you shall march around the city seven times, and the priests shall blow the trumpets. And it shall be that when they make a long
Trust	blast with the ram's horn, and when you **hear** the sound of the trumpet, all the people shall **shout** with a **great shout**; and the wall of the city will fall down flat, and the people will go up every man straight ahead."
Obey	Now Joshua rose early in the morning, and the priests took up the ark of the LORD. . . . they marched around the city once . . . and did so for six days.
Victory	On the seventh day they marched around seven times and the people **shouted** with a **great shout** and the wall fell down flat.

Selected verses from Joshua 6:1-22 NAS

Lord, when You tell me to do something that will eliminate my fears, may I have the faith and courage to be obedient. I trust that You are **with** me.

JUNE 7

If therefore your whole body is full of **light**,
with no dark part in it,
it shall be wholly illumined,
as when the lamp illumines you with its rays.
Luke 11:36 NAS

Lord, today I am feeling like this . . .

☺☺☺A smile is the window of your face
that tells people you are home.☺☺☺

JUNE 8

Consider it all **joy**, my brethren,
when you encounter various **trials,**
k n o w i n g
that the **testing** of your faith produces **endurance.**

And let endurance have its perfect result,
that you may be perfect and complete,
lacking in nothing.

But if any of you lacks **wisdom**,
let him ask of God,
who gives to all men generously
and without reproach,

and **it will be given to him.**

But let him ask in **faith** without any doubting,
for the one who doubts is like the surf of the sea
driven and tossed by the wind.

For let not that man expect that he will receive anything
from the Lord,
being a double-minded man, unstable in all his ways.

Blessed is a man who perseveres under trial;
for once he has been approved,
he will receive the **crown of life**,
which the Lord has promised
to those who love Him.

James 1:2-8, 12 NAS

JUNE 9

Meanwhile, Jesus and His disciples withdrew to the beach, followed by a huge crowd from all over Galilee, Judea, Jerusalem, Idumea, from beyond the Jordan River, and even from as far away as Tyre and Sidon.

> For the news about His miracles had spread far and wide and vast numbers came to see Him for themselves.

He instructed His disciples to bring around a boat and to have it standing ready to rescue Him in case He was crowded off the beach.

> For there had been many healings that day and as a result great numbers of sick people were crowding around Him, trying to touch Him.

And whenever those possessed by demons caught sight of Him they would fall down before Him shrieking,

> "You are the Son of God!"

But He strictly warned them not to make Him known.

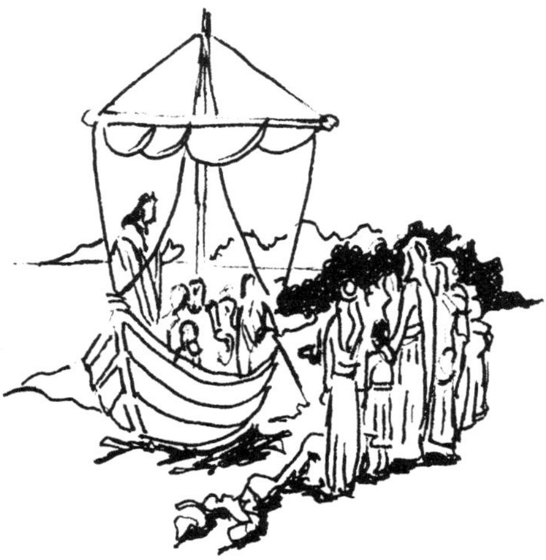

Mark 3:7-12 (TLB)

JUNE 10

When we came to Kansas City in June, 1990 to look for a house, we stayed with our son, David. For my morning devotions, I would go to his back porch where the view was to the east. As the sun rose at 5:30 each morning, God gave me a different message.

Day 1 A MOMENT IN TIME!
The birds are singing and the sky is aglow with shades of red everywhere. Quickly the beauty of the red sky fades and changes. Be ready for this moment in time.

Day 2 A NEW DAY DAWNING
Very cool breeze. Gentle daylight. No beautiful red sky. Slowly light arises.

Day 3 KEEP YOUR EYES ON THE LIGHT
A lone star in the sky. No brilliant pinks. Just light.

Day 4 SEARCH FOR THE STAR IN THE EAST AND FEEL THE HOLY SPIRIT BREEZE BLOWING
A new day of beauty is dawning. Warm.
Holy Spirit breeze blowing strong.

Day 5 THERE SHALL BE SHOWERS OF BLESSING
Rain all day. Praise the Lord for pouring blessings on us!

Day 6 GLORY! GLORY! DAWNS!
Bright SUN the morning after rain. A new day!

Day 7 LIGHT AND COLOR IN THE MIDST OF DARKNESS
Grey-blue clouds tinged with golden pink.
There is a balance of new light and pink
within the dark clouds.

JUNE 11

O P E N

W I D E

TO THE BLESSINGS

THAT GOD WANTS TO

SHOWER UPON YOU AND

YOUR LOVED ONES

JUNE 12

PASS IT ON

It only takes a spark to get a fire going,
And soon all those around can warm up in its glowing;
That's how it is with God's love, once you've experienced it;
You spread His love to everyone, you want to pass it on.

What a wondrous time is spring - when all the trees are budding,
The birds begin to sing, the flowers start their blooming;
That's how it is with God's love, once you've experienced it;
You want to sing, it's fresh like spring, you want to pass it on.

I wish for you, my friend, this happiness that I've found -
You can depend on him, it matters not where you're bound;
I'll shout it from the mountain top, I want my world to know;
The Lord of love has come to me, I want to pass it on.

Kurt Kaiser

JUNE 13

Admit fear of enemy

Jehoshaphat was afraid and turned his attention to seek the LORD; and proclaimed a fast throughout all Judah.

Prayer Meeting Lord's Prayer

So Judah gathered together to seek help from the LORD . . .
"O LORD, the God of our fathers, art Thou not God in the heavens? And art Thou not ruler over all the kingdoms of the nations? Power and might are in Thy hand so that no one can stand against Thee.

Praise for Past

Didst Thou not, O our God, drive out the inhabitants of this land before Thy people Israel, and give it to the descendants of Abraham Thy friend forever? And they lived in it and have built Thee a sanctuary there for Thy name, saying, "Should evil come upon us, the sword, or judgment, or pestilence, or famine,
we will stand before this house and before Thee (for Thy name is in **this house**) and
cry to Thee in our **distress**, and
Thou wilt hear and deliver us . . . .

Request

O our God, wilt Thou not judge them? For we are **powerless** before this great multitude who are coming against us; nor do we know what to do, **but our eyes are on Thee."**

Family Prayer

And all Judah was **standing before** the LORD, with their infants, their wives, and their children.

Hear God Speak

Then . . . the Spirit of the LORD came upon Jahaziel . . . and he said, "**Listen** . . . thus says the LORD to you,

Thru Others

Do not fear or be dismayed because of this great multitude, for the battle is not yours but God's.

Continued on June 14

JUNE 14

Plan of Action	Tomorrow go down against them. . . . You need not fight in this battle; station yourselves, stand and see the salvation of the LORD on your behalf. . . . **Do not fear or be dismayed,** . . . **for the LORD is with you."**
Accept Worship	And Jehoshaphat **bowed his head** . . . **worshiping** the LORD. . . . **stood up to praise** the LORD God of Israel, with a very loud voice. . . .
Obey Praise Tapes	"Listen to me . . . put your trust in the LORD your God, and you will be established." . . . And when they began singing and praising, the LORD set ambushes against . . .
Enemy Defeated	When Judah came to the lookout of the wilderness, they looked toward the multitude; and behold, they were corpses lying on the ground, and no one had escaped.
Blessings	And when Jehoshaphat and his people came to take their spoil, they found much among them, including goods, garments, and valuable things which they took for themselves, **more than they could carry**. And they were three days taking the spoil because there was so much.
To God be the Glory	Then on the fourth day they assembled in the valley . . . for there they blessed the LORD. . . . returning to Jerusalem with **joy**, for the LORD had made them to **rejoice** over their enemies. . . . So the kingdom of Jehoshaphat **was at peace**, for his **God gave him rest on all sides**.

2 Chronicles 20:3-30 NAS

JUNE 15

Beloved, I pray that in all respects

you may prosper and be in good health,

just as your soul prospers.

3 John 2 NAS

Lord, today I am feeling like this . . .

Don't pray for tasks equal to your strength,
but for strength equal to your tasks.

JUNE 16

Jesus now returned to the Sea of Galilee, and
climbed a hill and sat there.

And a vast crowd brought Him their lame, blind, maimed,
and those who couldn't speak, and many others,

and laid them before Jesus,

and **He healed them all.**

What a spectacle it was!

**Those who hadn't been able to say a word before
were talking excitedly,**

and those with missing arms and legs had new ones;

the crippled were walking and jumping around,

and those who had been blind were gazing about them!

The crowds just marveled,

and **praised the God of Israel.**

Matthew 15:29-31 (TLB). See also John 6:2-5.

JUNE 17

And immediately He made the disciples get into the boat,
and go ahead of Him to the other side,
while He sent the multitudes away.

And after He had sent the multitudes away,
He went up to the mountain by Himself to pray; and
when it was evening, He was there **alone**.

But the boat was already many stadia away from the land,
battered by the waves; for the **wind was contrary**.

And in the fourth watch (3:00 - 6:00 A.M.) of the night
He came up to them, **walking on the sea.**

And when the disciples saw Him walking on the sea, they were frightened,
saying, "It is a ghost!" And they cried out for fear.

But immediately Jesus spoke to them, saying,

"Take courage, it is I; do not be afraid."

And Peter answered Him and said, "Lord, if it is You, command me to come to you on the water."

And He said, *"Come!"* And Peter **got out of the boat,**
and walked on the water and came toward Jesus.

But seeing the wind, he became afraid, and beginning to sink,
he cried out, saying, "Lord, save me!"

And **immediately** Jesus stretched out His hand and
took hold of him, and said to him,

"O You of little faith, why did you doubt?"

And when they got into the boat, **the wind stopped**.

And those who were in the boat **worshiped** Him, saying,
"You are certainly God's Son!"

Matthew 14:22-33 NAS

JUNE 18

Mary remained with Elizabeth about three months and then returned home. Luke 1:56

How deeply moving is the story of Mary and Elizabeth sharing their awesome news together! God offers Mary an intimate friend with whom she can share what seems incommunicable. Elizabeth, like Mary, has experienced divine intervention and has been called to a response of faith. She can be with Mary in a way no one else possibly could. Amid an unbelieving, doubting, pragmatic and cynical world, two women meet each other and affirm in each other the promise given to them. For three months Mary and Elizabeth are linked and encourage each other to truly accept the motherhood given to them.

Neither had to wait in isolation. They could wait together and so deepen in each other their faith in God.

This surely is the rationale for Christian friendship and community. How can I ever let God's grace fully work in my life unless I live with people who can affirm it, deepen it and strengthen it? We cannot live this new life of faith alone. God does not want to isolate us when grace comes. Instead, God wants us to be linked, to be in new friendships and new communities - holy places where grace can grow to fullness and bear fruit.

Am I really trying to live my faith alone?
Is isolation hurting my faith?
Could I benefit from talking to a special Christian friend, a pastor, or should I join a small prayer or study group?

JUNE 19

GOD You who are a Father

You had to suffer, also

As You watched Your Son

die on the cross

You, who know the pain and helplessness

of seeing Your loved one suffer

HOLD ME in Your arms of love

while I cry out my pain

ROCK ME gently until

calm returns to my soul

SET ME back on my feet

to go back to my responsibility of caregiving

REFRESHED and RENEWED

because I've shared

with You, My heavenly Father

JUNE 20

WHOLE BODY HEALTH

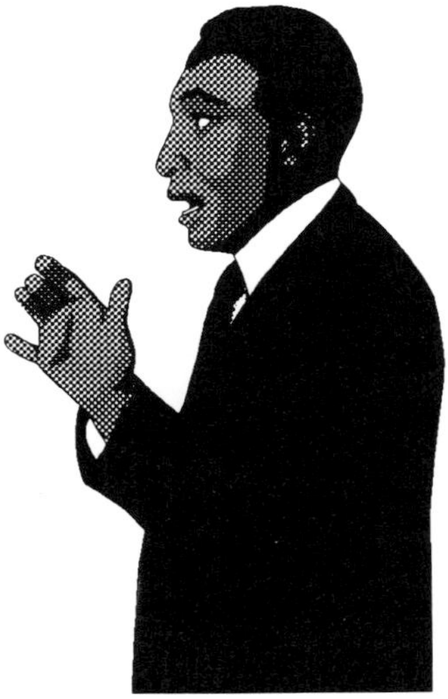

My son, give attention to my **words**;
Incline your **ear** to my sayings.
Do not let them depart from your **sight**;
Keep them in the midst of your **heart**.
For they are life to those who find them,
And **health** to all their **whole body**.
Watch over your **heart** with all diligence,
For from it flow the springs of life.
Put away from you a deceitful **mouth**,
And put devious **lips** far from you.
Let your **eyes** look directly ahead,
And let your **gaze** be fixed straight in front of you.
Watch the path of your **feet**,
And all your ways will be established.
Do not turn to the right nor to the left;
Turn your **foot** from evil.

Proverbs 4:20-27 NAS

JUNE 21

But He Himself would often slip away to the wilderness and pray.

Luke 5:16 NAS

Lord, today I am feeling like this . . .

If your trouble is long standing - try kneeling.

JUNE 22

The LORD will continually guide you,
And satisfy your desire in scorched places,
And give **strength** to your **bones;**
And you will be like a watered garden,
And like a spring of water whose waters do not fail.
Isaiah 58:11 NAS

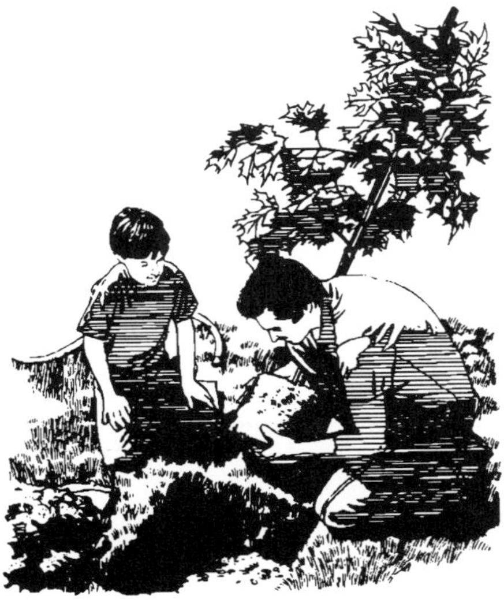

FUNNY BONE
Humor

BACKBONE
Courage

WISHBONE
Hope

KNEE BONE
Prayer

JUNE 23

Therefore, strengthen the **hands** that are weak

and the **knees** that are feeble,

and make straight paths for your **feet**,

so that the **limb which is lame**

may not be put out of joint,

but rather be **healed.**

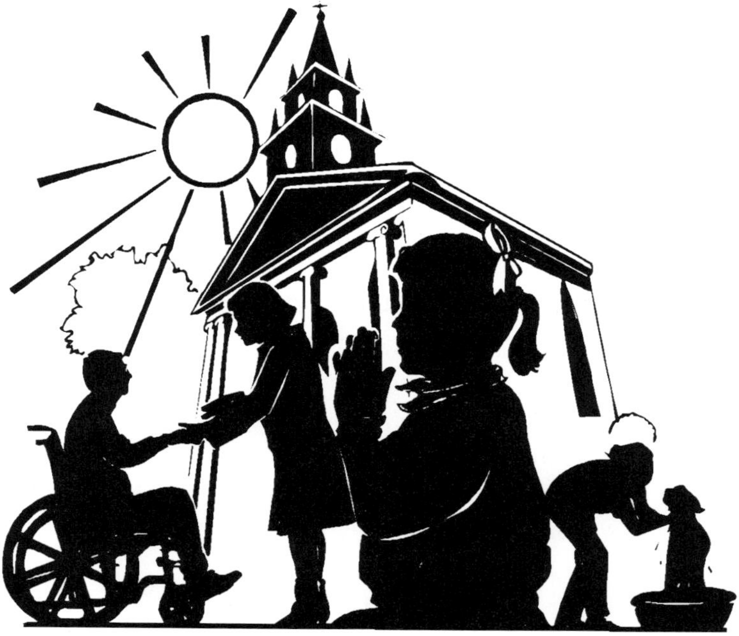

Hebrews 12:12-13 NAS

JUNE 24

When they arrived at the bottom of the hill,
a huge crowd was waiting for them.

A man came and knelt before Jesus and said,

> "Sir, have mercy on my son, for he is mentally deranged, and in great trouble, for he often falls into the fire or into the water; so I brought him to Your disciples, but they couldn't cure him."

Jesus replied,

> *"Oh, you stubborn, faithless people!*
> *How long shall I bear with you?*
> *Bring him here to me."*

Then Jesus rebuked the demon in the boy and it left him, and from that moment the boy was well.

Afterwards the disciples asked Jesus privately,

> "Why couldn't we cast that demon out?"
>
> *"Because of your little faith,"* Jesus told them.
> *"For if you had faith even as small as a tiny mustard seed*
> *you could say to this mountain,*
> *'Move!' and it would go far away.*
> ***Nothing would be impossible.***
> *But this kind of demon won't leave unless you have prayed and gone without food."*

Matthew 17:14-21 (TLB). See also Mark 9:17-29, Luke 9:37-42.

JUNE 25

And behold, an angel of the Lord suddenly appeared, and a light shone in the cell; and he struck Peter's side and roused him, saying, "Get up quickly."
And his chains fell off his hands.

Acts 12:7 NAS

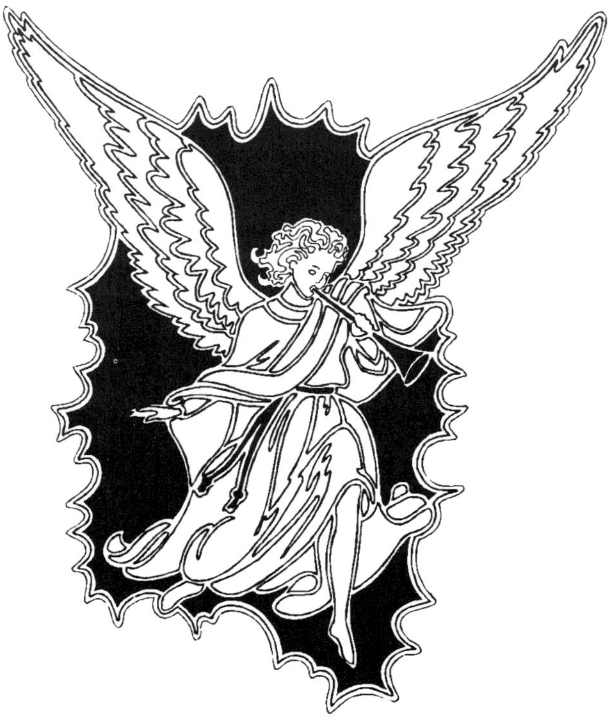

Then the devil left Him; and behold,
angels came and began to minister to Him.
Matthew 4:11 NAS

JUNE 26

Behold, I am going to send an **angel** before you to guard you along the way, and to bring you into the place which I have prepared.

Be on your guard before him and obey his voice;
do not be rebellious toward him . . .

But if you will truly **obey** his voice and **do** all that I say,
then I will be an enemy to your enemies and
an adversary to your adversaries.

For **My angel** will go before you and bring you in to
the land . . . and I will completely destroy them.

You shall not worship their gods, nor serve them,
nor do according to their deeds;
but you shall utterly overthrow them . . .

But you shall serve the LORD your God, and
He will **bless** your bread and your water; and

I will remove sickness from your midst. . . .

I will not drive them out before you in a single year,
that the land may not become desolate, and
the beasts of the field become too numerous for you.

I will drive them out before you little by little,

until you become fruitful and take possession of the land.

Selected verses from Exodus 23:20-30 NAS

JUNE 27

As I learned to play golf, I became aware of the similarities between the mechanics of the game of golf and my spiritual life.

Par Perfection/Goal
Score Measurement

Tee off Make first step toward goal
Long drives Major insights

Putts Small growth insights
Different clubs Worship, Prayer, Meditation, Bible Study, Serving, Memorization, Reading, Music

Foursome Friends are **with** me
God - Jesus - Holy Spirit - Me

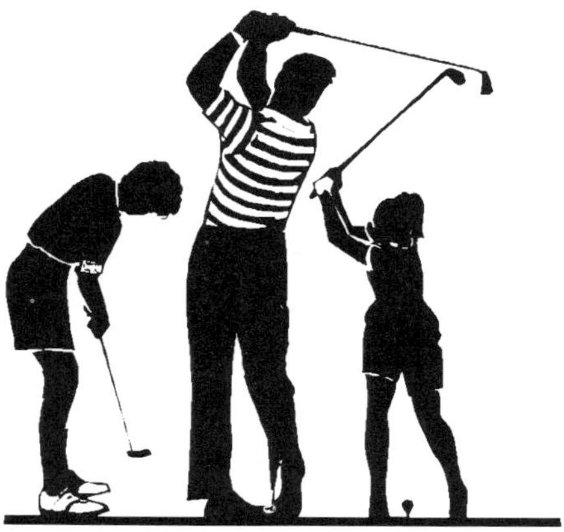

Continue on June 28

JUNE 28

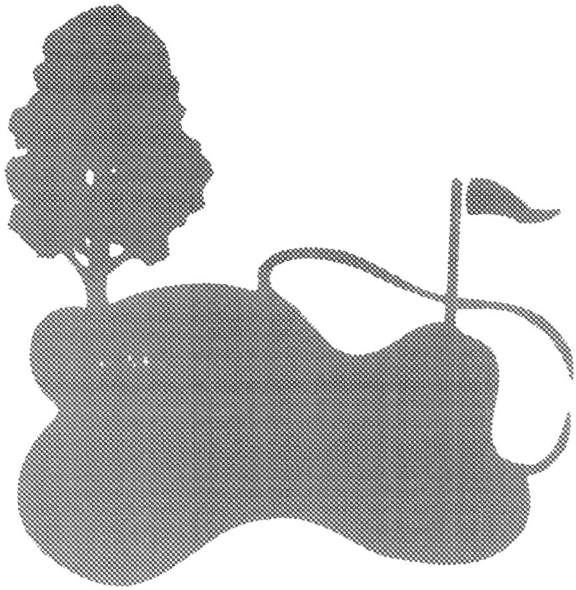

Shade & water & benches		Rest Times
Brag about scores/plays		Pride
	Course	Way is mapped out
	Holes	Complete one task then move on to the next one
Look for lost ball		Lost Souls
Out of bounds		Where I mess up (Sin)

JUNE 29

But as for me, I trust in Thee, O LORD,

I say, "Thou art my God."

My times are in Thy hand

Psalm 31:14-15 NAS

Lord, today I am feeling like this . . .

JUNE 30

And he (Mordecai) was bringing up . . . Esther, his uncle's daughter,
for she had neither father nor mother.
Now the young lady was beautiful of form and face,
and when her father and her mother died,
Mordecai took her as his own daughter.
Esther 2:7 NAS

Can a woman forget her nursing child,
And have no compassion on the son of her womb?
Even these may forget,
but I (God) will not forget you.
Behold, I (God) have inscribed you on the palms of My Hands . . .
Isaiah 49:15-16 NAS

For my father and my mother have forsaken me,
but the LORD will take me up.
Psalm 27:10 NAS

~~~~~~

Today is Betsy, our adopted daughter's, birthday.
She is our **chosen child** whom God sent to live with us when she was two and a half years old.

Opening our heart to love her has shown us another dimension of Our Heavenly Father's love for us.
He chooses to love us.
He is "there" for us.
He takes over for our natural parents.
He paid the price for us.
He rescues us from a life of misery and abandonment.
He gives us His full inheritance.
He personally brings us to the place in His family that He has prepared just for us.

~~~~~~

Father of Love, You are **with** us in this walk of suffering and caregiving. I praise You for choosing me to love. I nestle up into Your **big** Father Arms and let You hold me and comfort me.

JULY 1

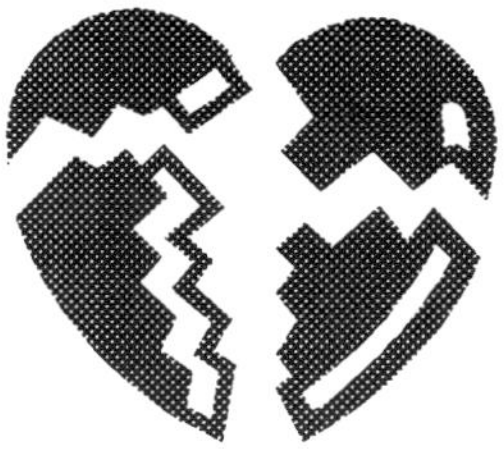

. . . I will give you a new heart
and put a new spirit with you;
and I will remove the heart of stone from your flesh
and give you a heart of flesh.

And I will put My Spirit within you
and cause you to walk in My statues,
and you will be careful to observe My ordinances.

And you will live in the land
that I gave to your forefathers;
so you will be My people,
and I will be your God.

Ezekiel 36:26-28 NAS

JULY 2

Jesus traveled around through all the cities and villages of that area, teaching in the Jewish synagogues and announcing the Good News about the Kingdom.

And wherever He went He healed people of every sort of illness.

And what pity He felt for the crowds that came,
because their problems were so great and
they didn't know what to do or where to go for help.
They were like sheep without a shepherd.

"The harvest is so great, and the workers are so few." He told His disciples. *"So pray to the one in charge of the harvesting, and ask Him to recruit more workers for His harvest fields."*

Matthew 9:35-37 (TLB)

JULY 3

But we have this treasure in earthen vessels,
that the surpassing greatness of the **power**
may be of God and not of ourselves;

we are **afflicted** in every way but not **crushed**;
perplexed but not **despairing**;
persecuted but not **forsaken**;
struck down but not **destroyed**;

always carrying about in the body the dying of Jesus,
that the **life** of Jesus also may be manifested in our body.

2 Corinthians 4:7-10 NAS

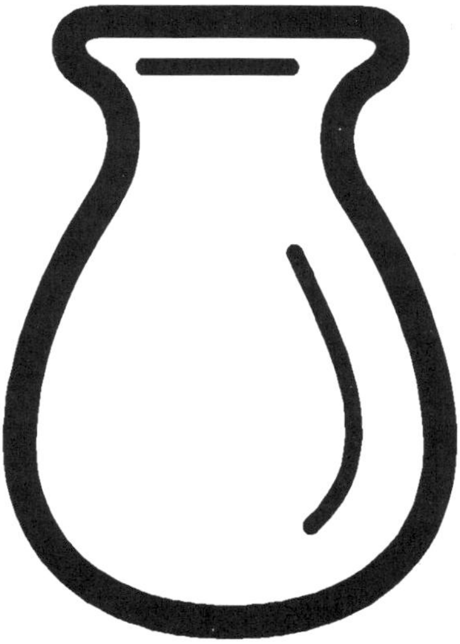

Lord, I feel like a **cracked pot**. Pour your healing oil into me and seal my cracks. Let **Your light shine** out of my cracks as **I pour myself** in loving service to my loved one.

JULY 4

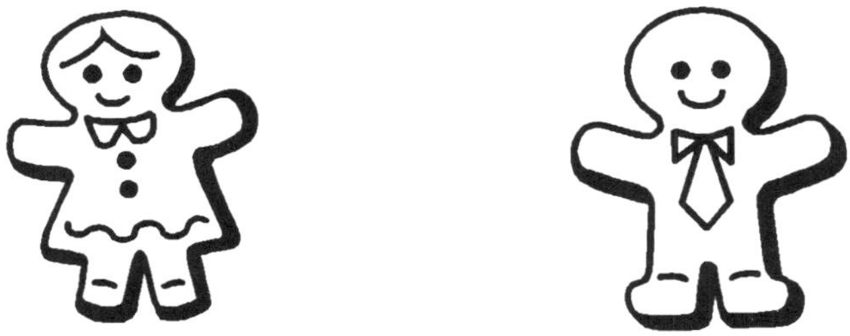

I feel like a cookie cutter trying to fulfill all my responsibilities. I am having to do so many things that I am not cut out to do. Feels like my own identity is getting cut off and reshaped.

spouse caregiver

parent nurse

banker sister child

gardener **I AM** housekeeper

brother friend

neighbor cook

grandparent employee

mechanic chauffeur

JULY 5

Choose for yourselves **today** whom you will serve . . .
as for me and my house, we will serve the LORD.
Joshua 24:15 NAS

THEIR ACTION	MY REACTION	MY CHOICE
She hates me	I can choose to hate her	I will choose **LOVE**
He is sad all all the time	I can choose to be sad	I will live with **JOY**
He is driving me crazy	I can choose retaliation	I will practice **PATIENCE**
Her words are hurtful	I can choose to be sassy	I will speak **KINDNESS**
He demands too much	I can choose to feel burdened	I will grow in **GOODNESS**
The world says "Leave him"	I can choose to leave	I will develop **FAITHFULNESS**
She is not her old self	I can choose to be angry	I will remember **GENTLENESS**
He makes me mad	I can choose to stay upset	I will nurture **SELF-CONTROL**

but the fruit of the Spirit is . . .
Galatians 5:22-23

JULY 6

For thus the LORD God, the Holy One of Israel, has said,

"In repentance and rest you shall be saved,

In quietness and trust is your strength."

Isaiah 30:15 NAS

Lord, today I am feeling like this . . .

____

____

____

____

____

____

____

____

____

____

____

____

The wise person turns a cross ✞ into a corsage ❀❀

JULY 7

HEALING TEAM MINISTRY

A day each week is needed for **rest**	Moses assembled all the congregation . . . For six days work may be done, but on the seventh day you shall have a holy day, a sabbath of complete rest to the LORD . . .
Heart for giving material things	Take from among you a contribution to the LORD; whoever is of a willing heart, let him bring it as the LORD'S contribution: gold, silver, bronze, blue . . . material, fine linen, goats' hair, rams' skins, . . . oil for lighting, spices for the anointing oil, . . . onyx stones . . .
Heart of craftsman	And let every skillful man among you come, and make all that the LORD has commanded: the tabernacle, . . . ark, . . . table, . . . lampstand, . . . altar, hangings, . . . woven garments . . .
Spirit stirs the heart	And everyone whose heart stirred him and everyone whose spirit moved him came and brought the LORD'S contribution for the work of the tent of meeting . . .
Coordinator of all	See, the LORD has called by name Bazalel . . . and He has filled him with the Spirit of God, in wisdom, in understanding and in knowledge and in all craftsmanship . . .
Teachable	He also has put in his heart to teach . . . He has filled them with skill to perform every work . . .
God provides all needs	For the material they had was sufficient and more than enough for all the work, to perform it.

Selected verses from Exodus 35-36:7 NAS

Lord, lead me to those medical personnel, pastors, support group leaders, pray-ers, friends, ministry teams who can help me with caregiving.

JULY 8

SANCTIFYING AND PERFECTING GRACE

454 Open My Eyes, That I May See

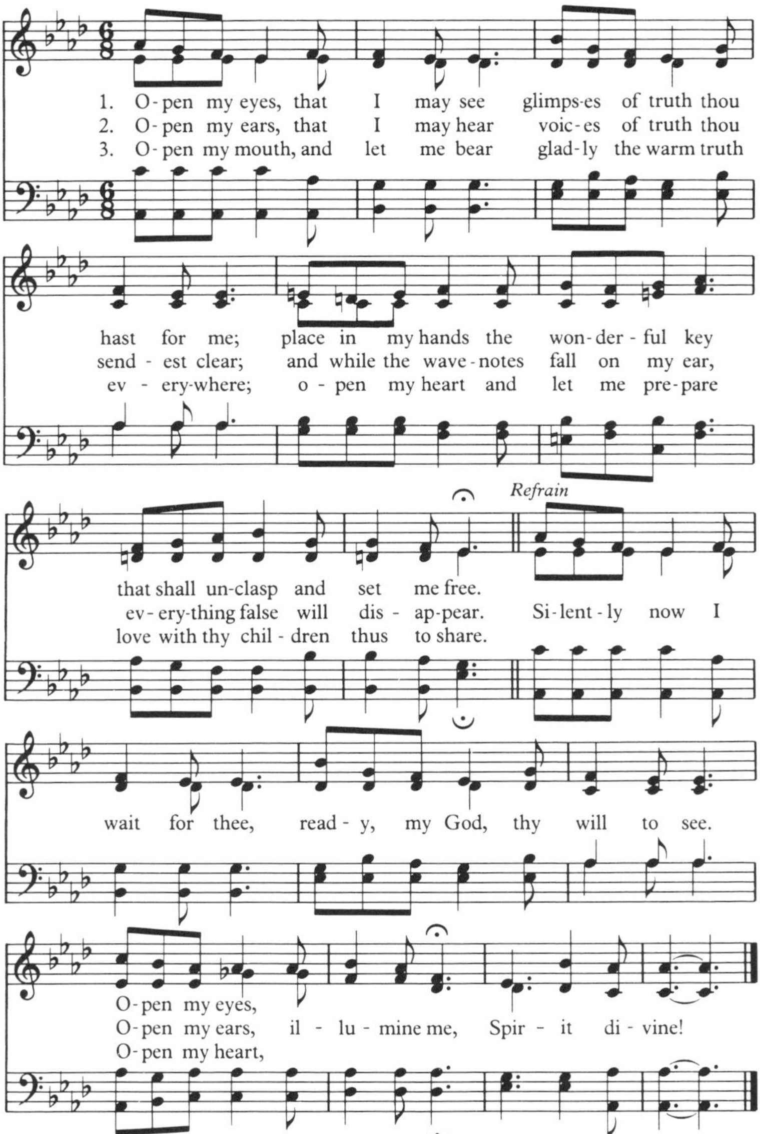

1. O-pen my eyes, that I may see glimps-es of truth thou
2. O-pen my ears, that I may hear voic-es of truth thou
3. O-pen my mouth, and let me bear glad-ly the warm truth
hast for me; place in my hands the won-der-ful key
send-est clear; and while the wave-notes fall on my ear,
ev-ery-where; o-pen my heart and let me pre-pare
that shall un-clasp and set me free.
ev-ery-thing false will dis-ap-pear.
love with thy chil-dren thus to share.
Refrain
Si-lent-ly now I
wait for thee, read-y, my God, thy will to see.
O-pen my eyes,
O-pen my ears, il-lu-mine me, Spir-it di-vine!
O-pen my heart,

WORDS: Clara H. Scott, 1895
MUSIC: Clara H. Scott, 1895

OPEN MY EYES
88.98 with Refrain

JULY 9

After Jesus had finished this address,
He left Galilee and circled back to Judea
from across the Jordan River.

Vast crowds followed Him,

and He **healed** their sick.

Matthew 19:1, 2 (TLB)

JULY 10

For we do not have a high priest who cannot
sympathize with our weaknesses,
but one who has been tempted in all things as we are,
yet without sin. (Jesus)

Let us therefore draw near with confidence
to the **throne of grace**,
that we may receive mercy and
may find grace to help in time of need.

Hebrews 4:15,16 NAS

JULY 11

When you walk through a storm,

Hold your head up high

And don't be afraid of the dark.

At the end of the storm

Is a golden sky

And the sweet silver song

of a lark. . . .

Walk on,

Walk on,

With hope in your heart,

And you'll never walk alone,

You'll never walk alone!

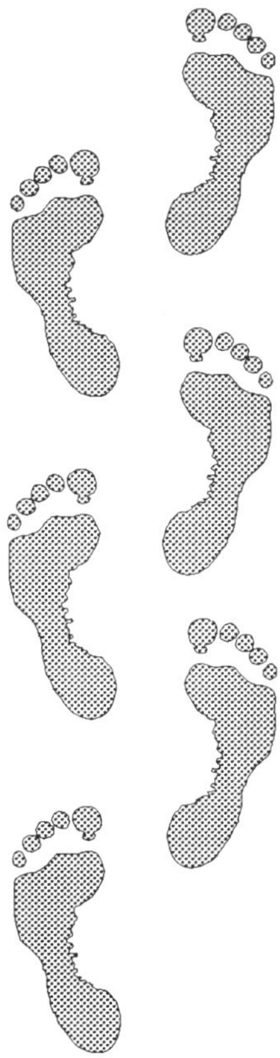

Lyric excerpts of "You'll Never Walk Alone"
by Richard Rodgers and Oscar Hammerstein II

Be strong and courageous,
do not be afraid or tremble at them,
for the Lord your God is the one
who goes **with** you.
He will not fail you or forsake you.
Deuteronomy 31:6 NAS

JULY 12

Do you know what makes me mad?

poison water

Poison water coming into our city,

that's what makes me mad!!

To capture a fortified city, an enemy only has to poison the water source coming into the city.

Do you want to know what the poison water is that is coming into our city?

Television	Magazines	Videos
Commercials	Newspapers	Music
Lotteries	Prize Contests	Movies
Gambling	Pornography	Abortion

and any other thing that pollutes our minds, spirits, and emotions.

From computers we have learned

garbage in **garbage out**

Whatever we put into our children's and our minds is what will come out in actions throughout our whole lives.

We tell our kids **"Just say no"**

But what are we telling them to **just say yes** to?

The gift of **love** we must give is to work hard to clean up the **poison water** in our lives and show our kids the

Clean, Living, Life-Giving Water they can say **"Yes"** to.

The following books give God's view of cities.
Reading them fills our minds with fresh "living water."

In His Steps, Charles Shelton
What happens to a town when the people ask in their daily life, "What would Jesus do?"

This Present Darkness, Frank Pereitti
The battle above and in a town between the forces of darkness and God's angels.

Joshua, Joseph F. Girzone
What happens to a town when a new man moves into the town.

DoorPosts, Timothy Botts
Scripture calligraphy that puts God's word on the **doorpost** of our heart homes.

JULY 13

. . . A time to be silent,

and a time to speak . . .

Ecclesiastes 3:7

Lord, today I am feeling like this . . .

Listen and **silent** have the same letters.

JULY 14

But Moses said to the people,

Have faith	"**Do not fear!** Stand by and see the salvation of the LORD which He will accomplish for you **today**; for the Egyptians whom you have seen today, you will never see them again forever.
Wait	The LORD will fight for you while you **keep silent**."
	Then the LORD said to Moses,
Obey	"Why are you crying out to Me? Tell the sons of Israel to go **forward**. And as for you,
Detail orders	lift up your staff and stretch out your hand over the sea and divide it and the sons of Israel shall go **through** the midst of the sea on dry land." . . .
God sends help	And the **angel** of God, who had been going before the camp of Israel, moved and went behind them; and the pillar of cloud moved from before them and stood behind them. . . .
God is faithful to His promise	And the sons of Israel went **through** the midst of the sea on dry land, and the waters were like a wall to them on their right hand and on their left.

Selected verses from Exodus 14:13-22 NAS

Lord, teach me to follow your leadership **through** this trouble, not around it. I am willing, Lord, to march forward, not do an about-face.

JULY 15

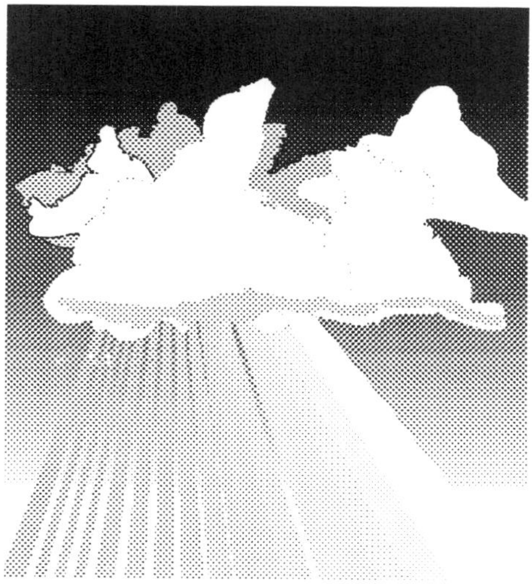

Jesus said,

"Peace I leave with you;

My peace I give you.

I do not give to you as the world gives.

Do not let your hearts be troubled

and do not be afraid."

John 14:27 NIV

JULY 16

As Jesus and the disciples left the city of Jericho,
a vast crowd surged along behind.

Two blind men were sitting beside the road and
when they heard that Jesus was coming that way,
they began shouting,

"Sir, King David's Son, have mercy on us!"

The crowd told them to be quiet,

but they only yelled the louder.

When Jesus came to the place where they were
He stopped in the road and called,

"What do you want me to do for you?"

"Sir," they said, "we want to see!"

Jesus was moved with pity for them

and **touched** their eyes.

And **instantly** they could see,

and **followed** Him.

Matthew 20:29-34 (TLB). See also Mark 10:46-52, Luke 18:35-43.

JULY 17

No, for the Scriptures tell us that for His sake we must be ready to face death at every moment of the day - we are like sheep awaiting slaughter; but despite all this, overwhelming **victory** is ours through Christ who loved us enough to die for us. For I am convinced that nothing can ever separate us from His love.

death can't

life can't

angels won't

all the powers of hell can't

our fears for today

our worries for tomorrow

where we are - high above the sky

or in the deepest ocean

NOTHING

will ever be able to separate us from
the love of God
demonstrated by our Lord Jesus Christ
when He died for us.

Romans 8:36-39 (TLB)

JULY 18

My Heart

Shield of Faith

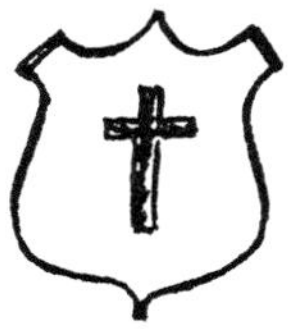

Arrow of satan's lie
Little truth on point

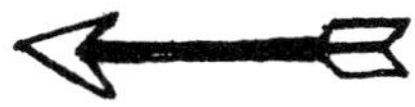

. . . taking up

the **shield of faith**

with which you will be able

to **extinguish** all the

flaming missiles of the evil one.

Ephesians 6:16 NAS

JULY 19

GOD SPEAKS THROUGH ROCKS

On an inner tubing trip on the Current River in southeast Missouri, I noticed bright red rocks in the crystal clear river. I began picking them up and noticed that after they were out of the water, they became dried out and were not as bright red. These rocks had many different shapes and indentations.

> We stay bright and shiny in God's **living water**
> with His 'Son-Light' on us.

Later that same summer we were at Atlantic Beach in North Carolina. Our favorite activity was to stand at the ocean's edge and pick up sea shells as they rolled in. I also began to pick up rocks. These rocks were grey and smooth as glass.

> Being tossed in and out and in and out, over time,
> smooths off the rough edges of our lives.

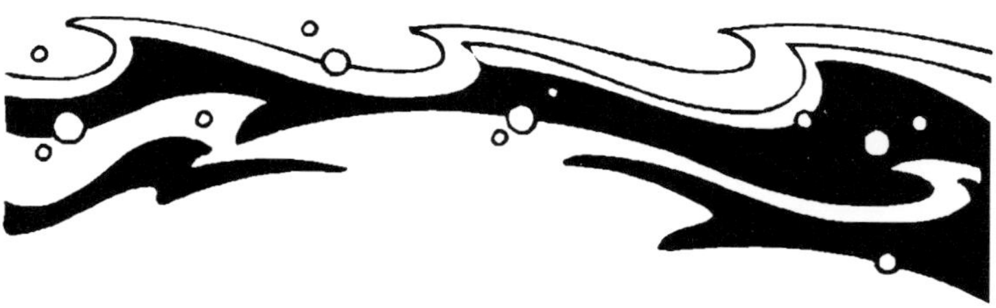

JULY 20

God was performing extraordinary miracles by the hands of Paul

Acts 19:11 NAS

Lord, today I am feeling like this . . .

Every miracle in the Bible begins with a problem.

JULY 21

O Lord, have mercy on me in my anguish.
My eyes are red from weeping;
my health is broken from sorrow.

I am pining away with grief;
my years are shortened,
drained away because of sadness.

My sins have sapped my strength;
I stoop with sorrow and with shame.
I am scorned by all my enemies
and even more by my neighbors and friends.
They dread meeting me and
look the other way when I go by.

I am forgotten like a dead man, like a broken and discarded pot.
I heard the lies about me,
the slanders of my enemies.
Everywhere I looked I was afraid,
for they were plotting against my life.

But I was trusting you, O Lord.
I said, "You alone are my God;
my times are in your hands.
Let your favor shine again upon your servant;
save me just because you are so kind!"

Hide your loved ones in the shelter of Your presence,
safe beneath Your hand . . .

Blessed is the Lord,
for He has shown me that His neverfailing love
protects me like the walls of a fort!

Psalm 31:9-16, 20, 21 (TLB)

JULY 22

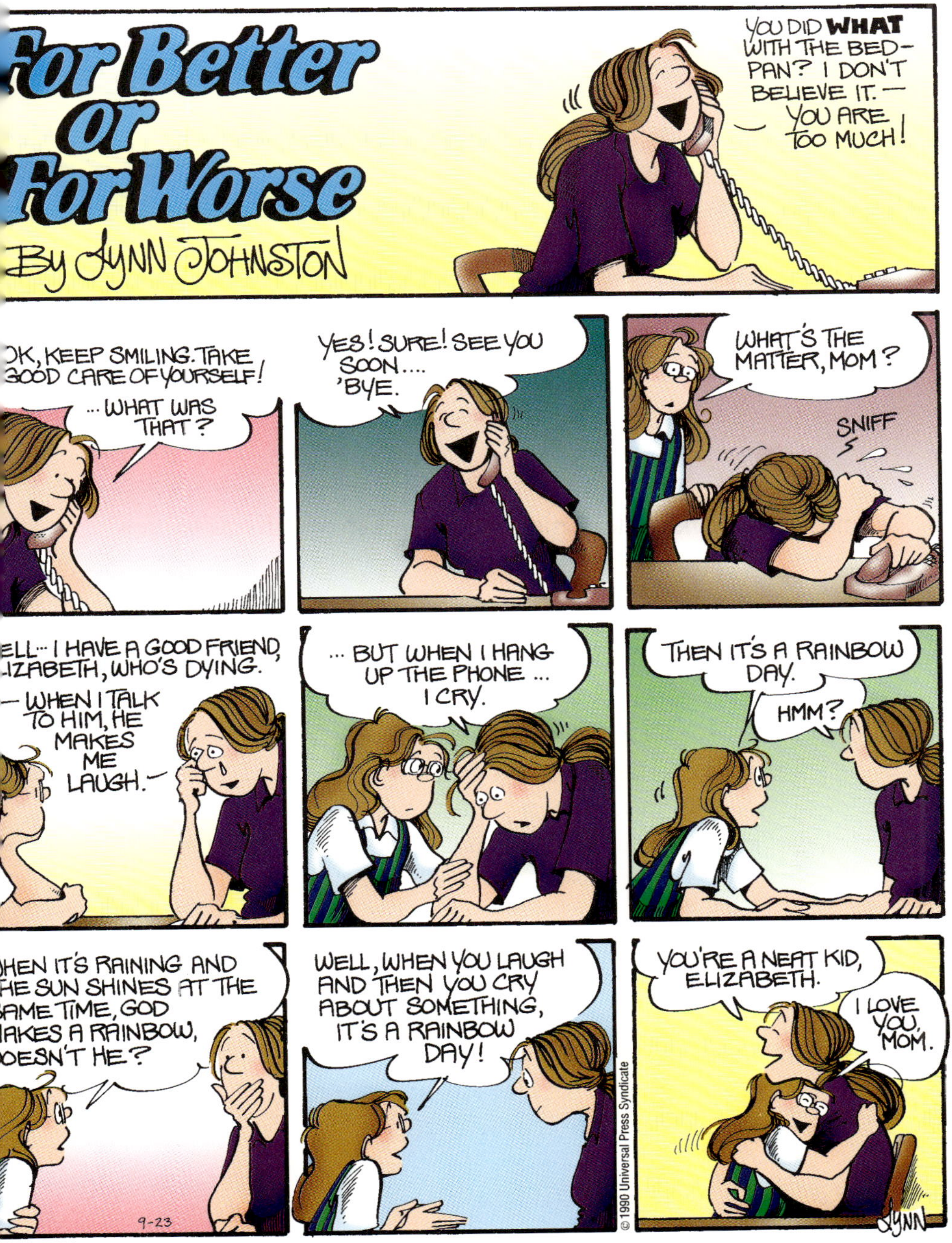
For Better or For Worse
By Lynn Johnston
YOU DID WHAT WITH THE BED-PAN? I DON'T BELIEVE IT. — YOU ARE TOO MUCH!
OK, KEEP SMILING. TAKE GOOD CARE OF YOURSELF!
... WHAT WAS THAT?
YES! SURE! SEE YOU SOON.... 'BYE.
WHAT'S THE MATTER, MOM?
SNIFF
ELL··· I HAVE A GOOD FRIEND, IZABETH, WHO'S DYING.
— WHEN I TALK TO HIM, HE MAKES ME LAUGH. —
... BUT WHEN I HANG UP THE PHONE ... I CRY.
THEN IT'S A RAINBOW DAY.
HMM?
HEN IT'S RAINING AND HE SUN SHINES AT THE AME TIME, GOD AKES A RAINBOW, OESN'T HE?
WELL, WHEN YOU LAUGH AND THEN YOU CRY ABOUT SOMETHING, IT'S A RAINBOW DAY!
YOU'RE A NEAT KID, ELIZABETH.
I LOVE YOU, MOM.
9-23
© 1990 Universal Press Syndicate
LYNN

JULY 23

JESUS SECOND TOUCH

When they arrived at Bethsaida,
some people brought a blind man to Him
and begged Him to touch and heal him.

Jesus took the blind man by the hand
and led him out of the village,
and spat upon his eyes,
and laid His hands over them.

"Can you see anything now?" Jesus asked him.

The man looked around.

"Yes!" he said, "I see men!
But I can't see them very clearly;
they look like tree trunks walking around!"

Then Jesus placed His hands over the man's eyes **again**
and as the man stared intently,
his sight was completely restored,
and he saw everything clearly,
drinking in the sights around him.

Jesus sent him home to his family.

"Don't even go back to the village first," He said.

Mark 8:22-26 (TLB). See also Matthew 9:27-31.

JULY 24

Do you not know that those who run in a race all run,
but only one receives the prize?

Run in such a way that you may win.

And everyone who competes in the games
exercises self-control in all things.
They then do it to receive a perishable wreath,
but we an imperishable.

Therefore I run in such a way,
as not without aim;
I box in such a way,
as not beating the air;
but I buffet my body and make it my slave,
lest possibly, after I have preached to others,
I myself should be disqualified.

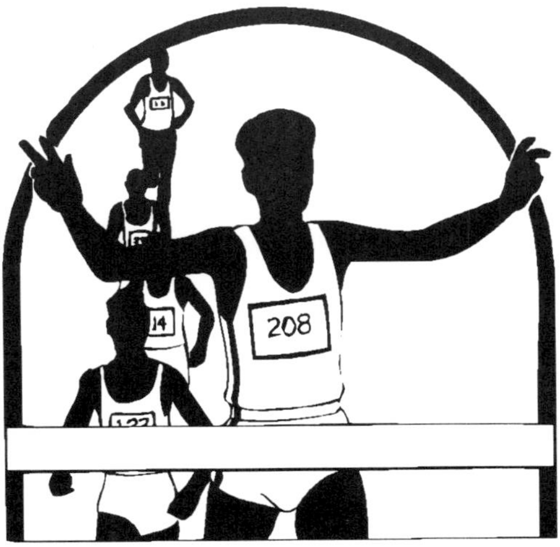

1 Corinthians 9:24-27 NAS

JULY 25

Hide your loved ones in the shelter of Your presence,
safe beneath your hand,
safe from all conspiring men.
Blessed is the Lord,
for He has shown me that His neverfailing love
protects me like the walls of a fort!
Psalm 31:20, 21 (TLB)

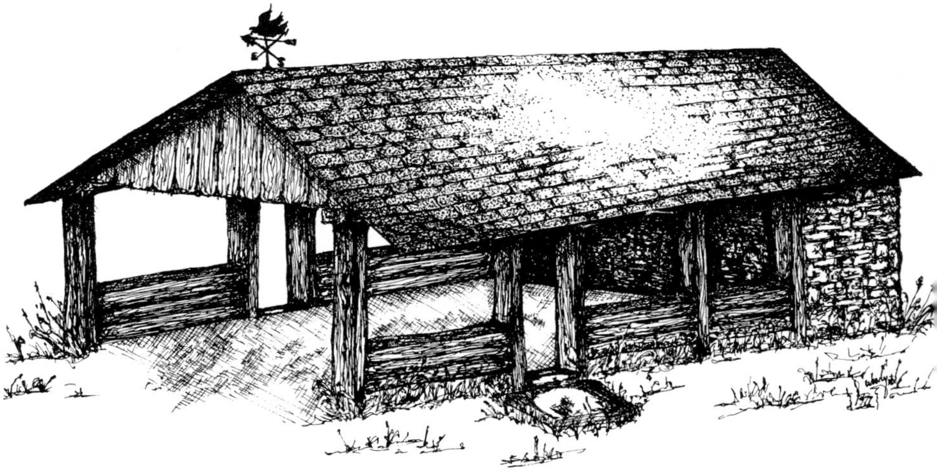

Drawing by Steve Wood of the Shelter House at
Woodland Acres, Greenfield Oh, 1977

JULY 26

Rejoice with those who rejoice, ☺

and weep with those who weep. ☹

Romans 12:15 NAS

TODAY I REJOICE FOR

1.

2.

3.

4.

5.

6.

7.

TODAY I WEEP FOR

1.

2.

3.

4.

5.

6.

7.

JULY 27

In 1990 as I drove behind the two U-Hauls for the 12-hour drive from Ohio to Kansas City, the following thoughts came to mind:

SHIFTING GEARS

Miles of highway   No radio
Time to **o p e n** my mind to God's thoughts
to **see** from His point of view,
looking down onto an interstate highway.

Here's a long stretch of flat land . . . things are going smoothly
Then comes a valley   and a **heavy** load to carry
from **here . . . . to . . . . there**
How do I do that?

I **decide** to get into the semi-truck,
have to **learn** to shift gears,
start out slow . . . get the feel of the road,
and trust in the vehicle and my driving skills.

It's a **l o n g** pull uphill;
others with lighter loads pass by quickly.

At the crest of the long hill is either
a quick descent or
another hill to climb or
a long, smooth, level road.

In each situation I have to **shift gears**.

Continued on July 28

JULY 28

I need a **rest stop**
a time to stretch a time to be refreshed.
Then back in my vehicle to continue toward my destination . . .
which is unseen to me at this moment,
but because I **trust** the road map
I **know** I will arrive at my goal.

Along the way are detours that change my route
and cause me delays.
Construction in progress makes a mess,
but the end result is a smoother ride
for those who will pass this way later.

The distance between my car and the two U-Hauls is bridged by communication over CB radios.
I am not alone.
I can give and receive instructions . . .
as long as we stay in close range and
have the radios turned on
Help is available . . . if I communicate my need.

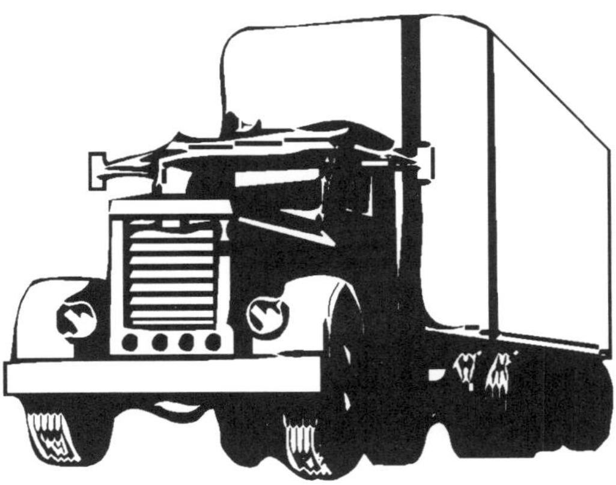

JULY 29

Come and hear,

all of you who reverence the Lord,

and **I will tell you what He did for me.**

For **I cried to Him for help,**

with **praises ready on my tongue.**

He would not have listened if I had not confessed my sins.

But He Listened!

He heard my prayer!

He paid attention to it!

Blessed be God who didn't turn away when I was praying,

and didn't refuse me His kindness and love.

Psalm 66:16-20 (TLB)

JULY 30

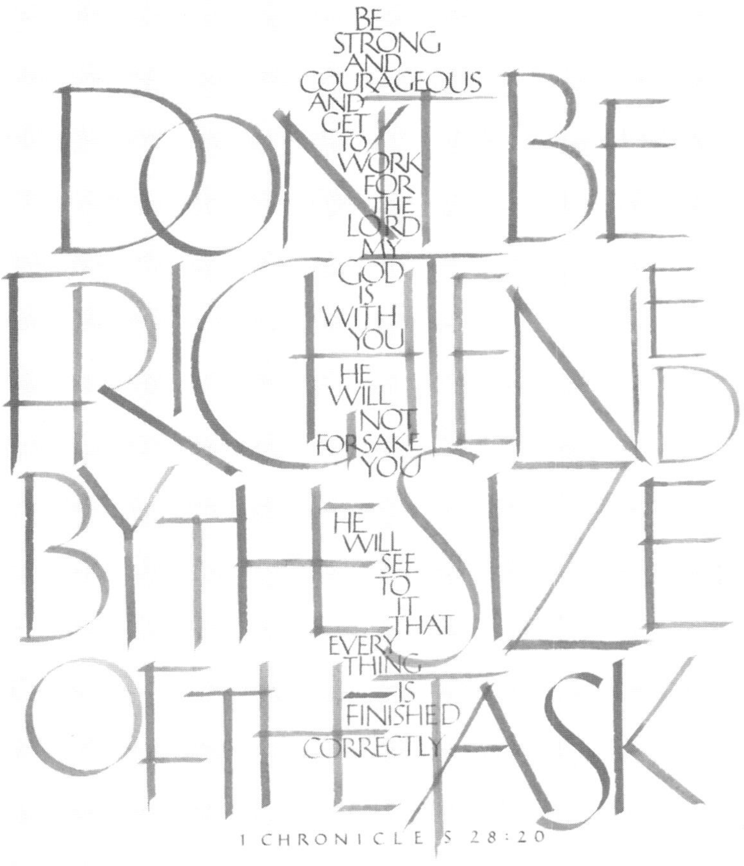
BE STRONG AND COURAGEOUS AND GET TO WORK FOR THE LORD MY GOD IS WITH YOU HE WILL NOT FORSAKE YOU HE WILL SEE TO IT THAT EVERYTHING IS FINISHED CORRECTLY
DON'T BE FRIGHTENED BY THE SIZE OF THE TASK
1 CHRONICLES 28:20

JULY 31

When they arrived on the other side of the lake,
in the country of the Gadarenes,
two men with demons in them met Him.

They lived in a cemetery and were so dangerous
that no one could go through that area.

They began screaming at Him,

"What do you want with us, O Son of God?
You have no right to torment us yet."

A herd of pigs was feeding in the distance, so the demons begged,

"If you cast us out, send us into that herd of pigs."

"All right," Jesus told them. *"Begone."*

And they came out of the men and entered the pigs,
and the whole herd rushed over a cliff and
drowned in the water below.

The herdsmen fled to the nearest city
with the story of what had happened,

and the entire population came rushing out to see Jesus,
and begged Him to go away and leave them alone.

Matthew 8:28-32 (TLB). Also see Mark 5:1-13,20 and Luke 8:26-39.

AUGUST 1

It is for **discipline** that you endure;
God deals with you as with sons;
for what son is there whom his father
does not discipline?

But if you are without discipline,
of which all have become partakers,
then you are illegitimate children and not sons.

Furthermore, we had earthly fathers to discipline us,
and we respected them;
shall we not much rather be subject to the
Father of spirits, and live?

For they disciplined us for a short time
as seemed best to them,
but He disciplines us for our good,
that we may share His holiness.

All discipline for the moment seems not to be joyful,
but sorrowful;
yet to those who have been trained by it,
afterwards it yields the peaceful fruit
of righteousness.

Hebrews 12:7-11 NAS

AUGUST 2

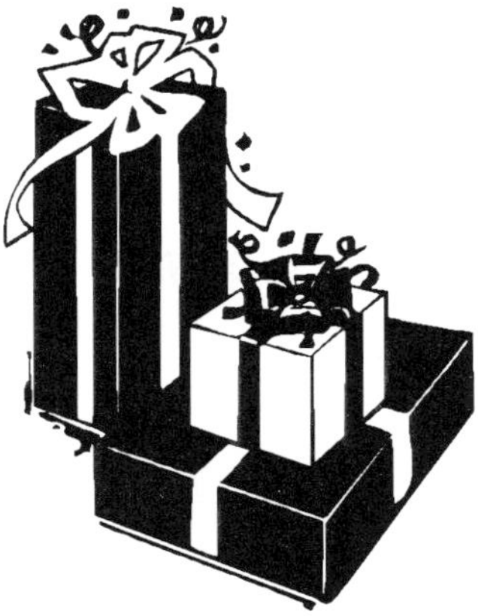

GOD,

give me grace to accept with

SERENITY

the things that cannot be changed,

COURAGE to change

the things which should be changed,

and the WISDOM

to distinguish the one from the other.

Reinhold Niebuhr

AUGUST 3

Let all bitterness and wrath and anger

and clamor and slander be put away from you,

along with all malice.

Ephesians 4:31 NAS

Lord, today I am feeling like this . . .

Anger is one letter short of **Danger**!

AUGUST 4

In Kansas City we moved into a house that was decorated and looked like it would have easy maintenance. It wasn't long before we found water in the basement under the upstairs bathroom tub.

I finally decided that the bathtub did not have grout around the edge next to the tile. I had never grouted before, and my attempt to do so was very sloppy. But I was satisfied that I had solved the problem.

No, there was still water coming into the basement. I called the plumber who had done the house inspection before we bought the house. He came and put a new drain trap in and showed me the clogged trap.

No, there was still water coming into the basement. I called another plumber, and he said we needed a new piece that opens and shuts the shower and its drain. So that was installed.

No, still water coming in. The plumber came back and said the plastic tile walls were not grouted. So I spent two weeks learning to grout tile walls, and I did the whole bathroom.

No, still water. My son and his wife analyzed the situation and finally realized that the water was seeping under the first grout job that I had done so poorly. So I took off the poorly done grout. By this time I had learned to grout correctly, and I regrouted the edge between the tub and the tile.

Problem solved!! I was right with my first diagnosis, only I had not done it correctly, and the experts I had consulted solved other problems but did not get to the root of the problem.

God showed me that trying to get to the root truth of Ron's medical condition was like this experience. I **know** what I **know** that I **know**. It just takes time and trial and error and lots of help from experts and family to get to the root of the problem.

AUGUST 5

DO NOT BE AFRAID

To Jeremiah — Jeremiah 1:8 NAS

"**Do not be afraid** of them,
For I am **with** you to deliver you,"
declares the LORD.

To Abraham — Genesis 15:1 NAS

. . . the word of the LORD came to Abram in a vision,
saying,
"**Do not fear**, Abram,
I am a shield to you;
Your reward shall be very great."

To Moses — Numbers 21:34 NAS

. . . the LORD said to Moses,
"**Do not fear** him,
for I have given him into your hand . . . "

To Daniel — Daniel 10:12,19 NAS

Then he (an angel) said to me,
"**Do not be afraid**, Daniel, for from the first day that
you set your heart on understanding this and
on humbling yourself before your God,
your words were heard, and
I have come in response to your words."
"O man of high esteem, **do not be afraid**.
Peace be with you;
take courage and be courageous!"

AUGUST 6

SWEET P'S: PRAYERS FROM GOD'S GARDEN

1. **Passion -** God's Love for you

   "You are altogether beautiful, My darling,
   And there is no blemish in you.
   You have made My heart beat faster, My sister, My bride;
   You have made My heart beat faster with a single glance of your eyes."
   Song of Solomon 4:7,9 NAS

2. **Purpose -**

   God has **saved** us, and **called** us with a **holy calling**, not according to our works, but according to His own **purpose** and grace which was granted us in Christ Jesus from all eternity.
   2 Timothy 1:9 NAS

3. **People -**

   They brought beds, basins, pottery, wheat, barley, flour, parched grain, beans, lentils, parched seeds, honey, curds, sheep, and cheese of the herd, for David and for the people who were with him, to eat; for they said, "The people are hungry and weary and thirsty in the wilderness." 2 Sam. 17:28,29 NAS

4. **Provision -**

   And my God shall supply **all your needs** according to His riches in glory in Christ Jesus. Philippians 4:19 NAS

5. **Peace -**

   Be anxious for nothing, but in everything by prayer and supplication with thanksgiving let your requests be made known to God.
   And the **peace of God**, which surpasses all comprehension, shall guard your heart and your mind in Christ Jesus.
   Philippians 4:6,7 NAS

6. **Power -**

   You shall receive **power** when the Holy Spirit has come upon you; and you shall be My witnesses . . . Acts 1:8 NAS

7. **Protection -**

   For **He will give His angels charge concerning you,**
   To guard you in all your ways. They will bear you up in their hands,
   Lest you strike your foot against a stone.
   Psalm 91:11,12 NAS

AUGUST 7

Jesus and His companions now arrived at the town of Capernaum and on Saturday morning went into the Jewish place of worship - the synagogue - where He preached.

The congregation was surprised at His sermon because He spoke as an authority, and didn't try to prove His points by quoting others - quite unlike what they were used to hearing!

A man possessed by a demon was present and began shouting,

"Why are you bothering us, Jesus of Nazareth -
have You come to destroy us demons?
I know who You are - the Holy Son of God!"

Jesus curtly commanded the demon to say no more
and to come out of the man.

At that the evil spirit screamed and
convulsed the man violently and left him.

Amazement gripped the audience and
they began discussing what had happened.

"What sort of new religion is this?" they asked excitedly.
"Why, even evil spirits obey His orders!"

The news of what He had done spread quickly
through that entire area of Galilee.

Mark 1:21-28 (TLB). See also Luke 4:33-36.

AUGUST 8

DO NOT BE AFRAID

To Mary — Luke 1:30 NAS

And the angel said to her,
"**Do not be afraid,** Mary;
for you have found favor with God."

To Shepherds — Luke 2:10 NAS

And the angel said to them,
"**Do not be afraid**; for behold,
I bring you good news of a great **joy**
which shall be for **all** the people;
for today in the city of David
there has been born **for you** a Savior,
who is Christ the Lord."

To Peter — Luke 5:10b NAS

And Jesus said to Simon,
"**Do not fear**,
from now on you will be catching men."

To Paul — Acts 27:23-26 NAS

"For this very night an angel of the God
to whom I belong and whom I serve stood before me,
saying, '**Do not be afraid,** Paul;
you must stand before Caesar; and behold,
God has granted you all those who are sailing with you.'
Therefore, keep up your courage, men, for I believe God,
that it will turn out exactly as I have been told."

AUGUST 9

Caregiving is like an ice tea pitcher.
It is an outpouring of self into another.
Just as the ice tea pitcher has to be refilled to be served again,
so, too, the caregiver has to be refilled by the Holy Spirit in
worship, rest, relaxation, and by friends and food.

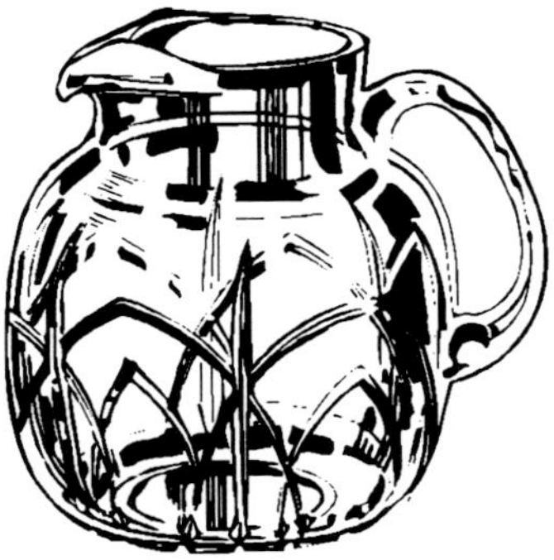

Lord, by an act of my will, I choose to open up to be refilled
with the fruits of the Spirit found in Galatians 5:22, 23:

love, joy, peace,
patience, kindness, goodness,
faithfulness, gentleness, and self-control.

And this I pray,
that your love may abound still more and more
in real knowledge and all discernment,
so that you may approve the things that are excellent,
in order to be sincere and blameless until the day of Christ;
having been filled with the fruit of righteousness
which comes through Jesus Christ,
to the glory and praise of God.

Philippians 1:9-11 NAS

AUGUST 10

. . . you are **precious** in My sight, . . .

you are honored

and I love you . . .

Isaiah 43:4 NAS

Lord, today I am feeling like this . . .

God Loves You, I Love You

AUGUST 11

If I want plants to grow
I must **let go** of the seeds
and let them fall to the ground
and be buried under the soil.

When potatoes are planted
an old potato with new "eyes"
is buried in the ground.
It becomes food for the new plant;
the new growth is hidden underground.

let go of the seeds
so they fall
and
are buried underground
then
roots and shoots form
and
new growth appears

I must die to my selfish desires, and let God cause new growth to begin **in** me and new fruit to come forth in my life.

. . . unless a grain of wheat falls into the earth and dies,
it remains by itself alone;
but if it dies,
it bears much fruit.

John 12:24 NAS

AUGUST 12

THREE PEOPLE DO THREE THINGS

Hezekiah became mortally ill.

I. **Isaiah** came to Hezekiah and said:

A. "Thus says the LORD, 'Set your house in order, for you shall die and not live.' "

B. **Immediately** the Word of LORD came to **Isaiah** to tell Hezekiah three things:

1. Lord heard his prayer
2. Saw his tears
3. Would heal him

On **the third day** Hezekiah was to go to the house of LORD (worship).

C. **Isaiah** gave Hezekiah practical (medical) advice:

1. "Take a cake of figs"
2. They took it and laid it on the boil
3. He recovered

II. **Hezekiah** did three things:

A. Turned his face to the wall
B. Prayed to LORD to remember his faithfulness
C. Wept bitterly

III. **God** will do three things for Hezekiah:

A. Add 15 years to his life
B. Deliver him and city from enemies
C. Defend city for His own sake

2 Kings 20:1-11 NAS. See also Isaiah 38:1-22.

AUGUST 13

TO SATAN'S

L I E

ADD

F AITH IN GOD

AND RECEIVE ETERNAL

L I F E

AUGUST 14

Several days later He returned to Capernaum,
and the news of His arrival spread quickly through the city.

> Soon the house where He was staying was so packed with visitors that there wasn't room for a single person more, not even outside the door.

And He preached the Word to them.

Four men arrived carrying a paralyzed man on a stretcher.

> They couldn't get to Jesus through the crowd,
> so they dug through the clay roof above His head
> and lowered the sick man on his stretcher,
> right down in front of Jesus.

When Jesus saw how strongly they believed that He would help,
Jesus said to the sick man,

> *"Son, your sins are forgiven!"*

But some of the Jewish religious leaders said to themselves as they sat there,

> "What? This is blasphemy! Does He think He is God?
> For only God can forgive sins."

Jesus could read their minds and said to them at once,

> *"Why does this bother you?*
> *I, the Messiah, have the authority on earth to forgive sins.*
> *But talk is cheap - anybody could say that.*
> *So I'll prove it to you by healing this man."*

Continued on August 15

AUGUST 15

Then, turning to the paralyzed man, He commanded,

> *"Pick up your stretcher and go on home,*
> *for you are healed!"*

The man jumped up,
took the stretcher,
and pushed his way through the stunned onlookers!

Then how they praised God.

> "We've never seen anything like this before!"
> they all exclaimed.

Mark 2:1-12 (TLB). See also Matthew 9:2-7, Luke 5:17-25.

Pretend this is a stretcher, and your loved one is lying on it. Write in the names of four family members or friends who are helping you carry your loved one. If you do not have any family or friends to help you, remember Jesus' words in John 14:16, *"And I will ask the Father, and He will give you another Helper that He may be with you forever . . . "*

Practically, ask God where you can reach out to a church, a support group, or neighbors for help. No one can carry the burden alone. Write your loved one's name on the stretcher.

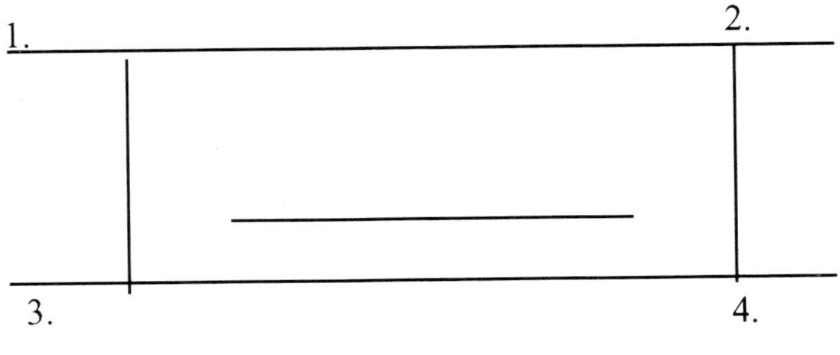

AUGUST 16

For **I have learned to be content**
in whatever circumstances I am.

I know how to get along with humble means,
and I also know how to live in prosperity;

In **any** and **every** circumstance
I have learned the secret of being filled and going hungry,

both of having abundance and suffering need.

I CAN DO

ALL THINGS

THROUGH HIM WHO

STRENGTHENS ME

Philippians 4:11-13 NAS

AUGUST 17

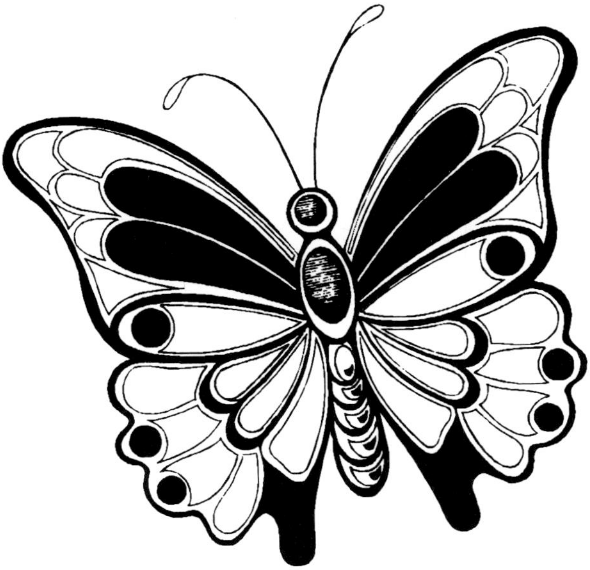

Jesus said,

"If you abide in My word,

then you are truly disciples of Mine;

and you shall know the truth, and

the truth shall make you free."

John 8:31,32 NAS

AUGUST 18

There is no fear in love;

but perfect love casts out fear . . .

1 John 4:18 NAS

Lord, today, I am feeling like this . . .

TODAY I choose to live in God's love and not in fear.

AUGUST 19

I will praise you, Lord,
for you have saved me from my enemies.
You refuse to let them triumph over me.

O Lord my God,
I pleaded with you, and you gave me my health again.
You brought me back from the brink of the grave,
from death itself, and here I am alive!

Oh, sing to Him you saints of His;
give thanks to His Holy Name.
His anger lasts a moment; His favor lasts for life!

Weeping may go on all night,
but in the morning there is **joy**.

In my prosperity I said,
"This is forever; nothing can stop me now!
The Lord has shown me His favor.
He has made me steady as a mountain."

Then, Lord, You turned Your face away from me
and cut off Your river of blessings.
Suddenly my courage was gone;
I was terrified and panic-stricken.
I cried to You, O Lord: oh, how I pled:

"What will you gain, O Lord, from killing me?
How can I praise You then to all my friends?
How can my dust in the grave speak out and
tell the world about your faithfulness?
Hear me, Lord; oh, have pity and help me."

Then He turned my sorrow into **joy**!
He took away my clothes of mourning
and gave me gay and festive garments to rejoice in
so that I might sing glad praises to the Lord
instead of lying in silence in the grave.

O Lord my God,
I will keep on thanking You forever!

Psalm 30 (TLB)

AUGUST 20

All the way my Savior leads me. What have I to ask beside? Can I doubt His tender mercy, Who through life has been my guide?

AUGUST 21

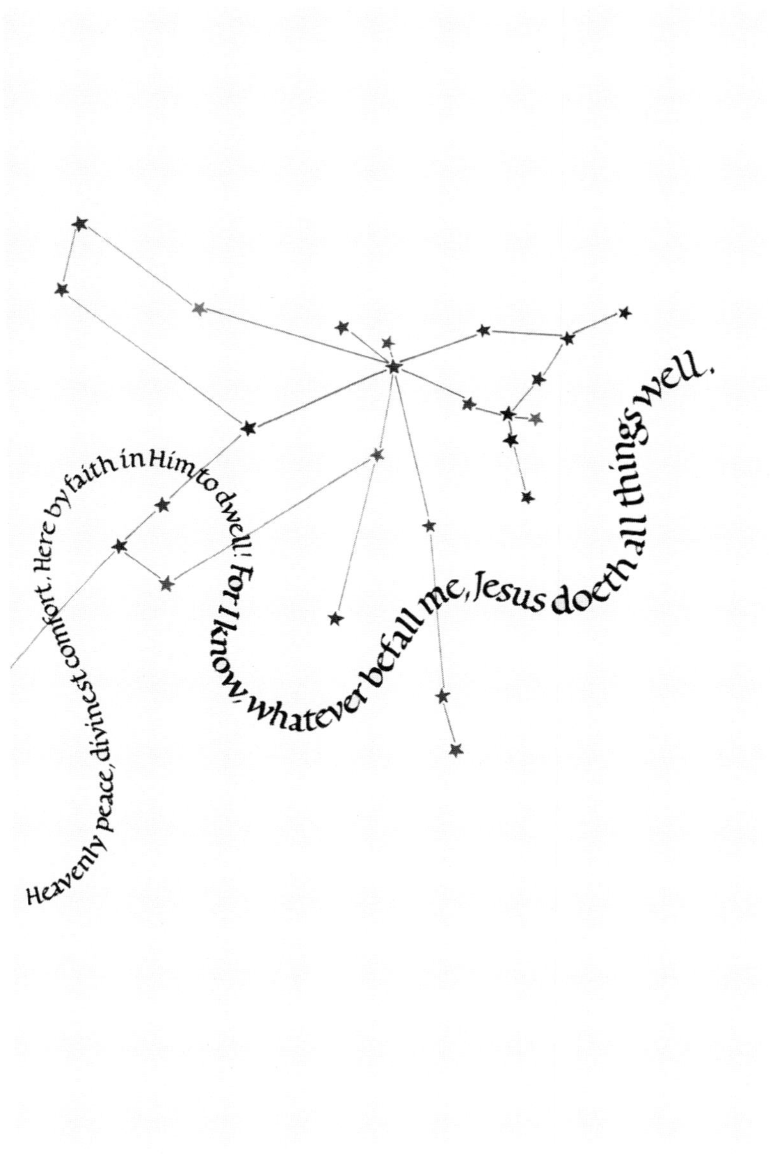
Heavenly peace, divinest comfort, Here by faith in Him to dwell! For I know, whatever befall me, Jesus doeth all things well.

AUGUST 22

S O R R Y

L O R D !!

These are ways I have hurt you, Lord.
I receive Your forgiveness for these actions.

1.____

2.____

3.____

4.____

If we **confess** our sins,
He is faithful and righteous to forgive us our sins
And to cleanse us from all unrighteousness.
1 John 1:9 NAS

AUGUST 23

From Tyre He went to Sidon,
then back to the Sea of Galilee
by way of the Ten Towns.

A deaf man with a speech impediment
was brought to Him,
and everyone begged Jesus to lay His hands
on the man and heal him.

Jesus led him away from the crowd and
put His fingers into the man's ears, then
spat and touched the man's tongue with the spittle.

Then, looking up to heaven, He sighed and commanded,

"O P E N!"

Instantly the man could hear perfectly and speak plainly!

Jesus told the crowd not to spread the news,
but the more He forbade them,
the more they made it known,
for they were overcome with utter amazement.

Again and again they said,

"Everything He does is wonderful;
He even corrects deafness and stammering!"

Mark 7:31-37 (TLB)

AUGUST 24

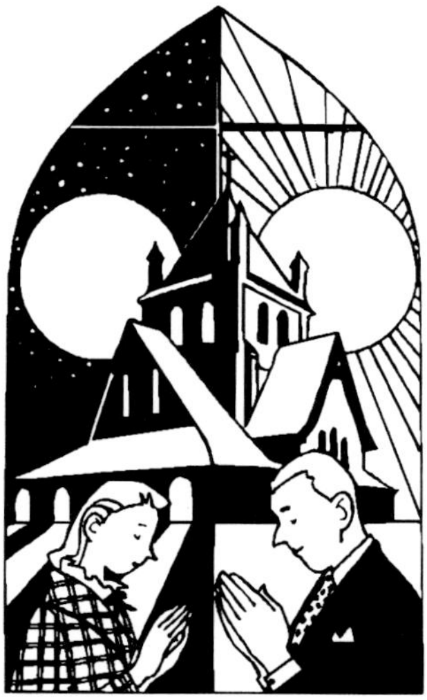

As for me,
I shall call upon God,
and the LORD will save me.
Evening and morning and at noon,
I will complain and murmur,
and He will hear my voice.
He will redeem my soul in peace
from the battle which is against me,
for they are many who strive with me.
Psalm 55:16-18 NAS

Even those I will bring to My holy mountain,
and make them joyful in
My house of prayer. . . .
For My house will be called a
house of prayer for all peoples.
Isaiah 56:7 NAS

AUGUST 25

But I am among you as the one who serves.

And you are those who have stood by Me in My trials.

Luke 22:27, 28 NAS

Lord, today I am feeling like this . . .

Life is like tennis. Learn to serve best.

AUGUST 26

. . . brought

beds	basins	pottery	wheat
barley	flour	beans	lentils
honey	curds	sheep	cheese
parched grain		parched seeds	

for David and for the people who were with him,

to eat;

for they said,

"The people are hungry and

weary and

thirsty

in the **wilderness**."

2 Samuel 17:28, 29 NAS

Who can you count on for practical help in your daily needs and responsibilities? List them, call them, ask for help.

1.____

2.____

3.____

AUGUST 27

We give **thanks** to God,
the Father of our Lord Jesus Christ,
praying always for you,
since we heard of your faith in Christ Jesus
and the **love** which you have for all the saints;
because of the **hope** laid up for you in heaven,
of which you previously heard in the word of truth,
the gospel . . .

For this reason also, since the day we heard of it,
we have not ceased to pray for you
and to ask that

1. You may be **filled** with the knowledge of His will
   in all spiritual wisdom and understanding,
2. So that you may **walk** in a manner worthy of the Lord,
3. To **please** Him in all respects,
4. **Bearing fruit** in every good work
5. And **increasing** in the knowledge of God;
6. **Strengthened** with all **power**,
   according to His glorious might,
   for the attaining of all steadfastness and patience;
7. **Joyously** giving **thanks** to the Father,
   who has qualified us to share in the
   inheritance of the saints in **light**.

For He delivered us from the domain of darkness,
and transferred us to the kingdom of His beloved Son,
in whom we have redemption,
the forgiveness of sins.

Colossians 1:3-5, 9-14 NAS

AUGUST 28

As Jesus was leaving her home,
two blind men followed along behind, shouting,

"O Son of King David, Have mercy on us."

They went right into the house where He was staying,
and Jesus asked them,

*"Do you **believe** I can make you see?"*

"Yes, Lord," they told Him, "we do."

Then He **touched** their eyes and said,

"Because of your faith it will happen."

And **suddenly they could see!**

Jesus sternly warned them not to tell anyone about it,
but instead they spread His fame all over the town.

Matthew 9:27-31 (TLB). See also Mark 8:22-26.

AUGUST 29

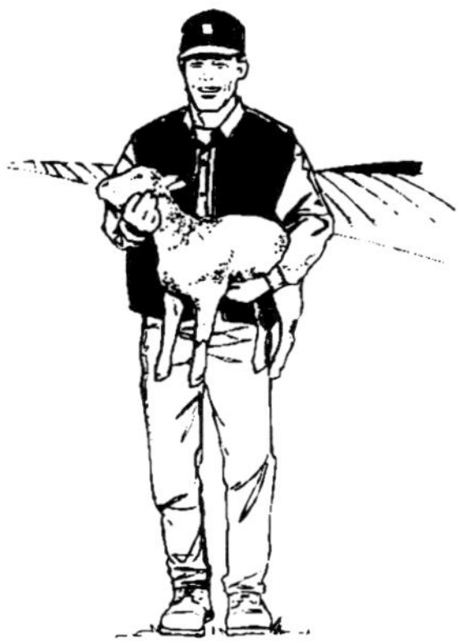

Personalize with your or your loved one's name the

TWENTY THIRD PSALM from NIV

The LORD is _______________ shepherd,
_______________shall not be in want.
He makes ________________lie down in green pastures,
He leads ________________beside quiet waters,
He restores ________________ soul.
He guides ___________in paths of righteousness for His name's sake.
Even though _______________walks **through** the
valley of the shadow of death, ________________will fear no evil,
For You are **with** ________________;
Your rod and staff, they comfort _______________.
You prepare a table before ________________
in the presence of _______________enemies.
You anoint ________________head with oil;
________________cup overflows.
Surely goodness and love will follow _______________
all the days of _______________ life,
and _______________ will dwell in the House of the LORD,
forever!!

AUGUST 30

Not long afterwards Jesus went with His disciples to the village of Nain, with the usual great crowd at His heels.

A funeral procession was coming out
as He approached the village gate.

The **boy who had died** was the only son of his widowed mother, and many mourners from the village were with her.

When the Lord saw her, His heart overflowed with sympathy.

"Don't cry!" He said.

Then He walked over to the coffin and **touched** it,
and the bearers stopped.

"Laddie," he said, *"come back to life again."*

Then the boy sat up and began to talk to those around him!

And Jesus gave him back to his mother.

Luke 7:11-15 (TLB)

AUGUST 31

. . . For I will turn their **mourning** into **joy**,

And will **comfort** them,

And give them **joy** for their sorrow.

Jeremiah 31:13 NAS

Lord, today I am feeling like this . . .

SEPTEMBER 1

And by the river on its bank,
on one side and on the other,
will grow all kinds of trees for food.
Their leaves will not wither,
and their fruit will not fail.

They will bear every month
because their water flows from the sanctuary,
and their fruit will be for food
and their **leaves for healing**.
Ezekiel 47:12 NAS

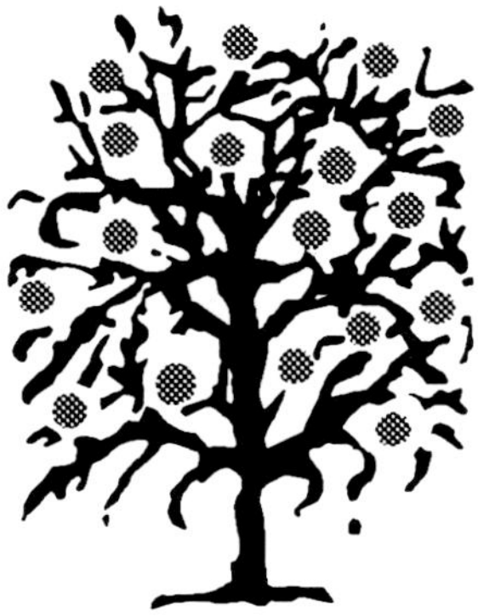

And he showed me a river of the water of life,
clear as crystal,
coming from the throne of God and of the Lamb,
in the middle of its street.

And on either side of the river
was the tree of life,
bearing twelve kinds of fruit,
yielding its fruit every month;
and the **leaves of the tree were for healing of the nations.**
Revelation 22:1-2 NAS

SEPTEMBER 2

Do not call to mind the former things,
Or ponder the things of the past.

Behold I will do **something new**,
Now it will **spring** forth;
Will you not be aware of it?

I will even make a **roadway in the wilderness,**
rivers in the desert.

The beasts of the field will glorify Me;
The jackals and the ostriches;

Because I have given **waters in the wilderness**
And **rivers in the desert**,
To give drink to **My chosen people.**

The people whom I formed for Myself,
will declare **My praise**.

Isaiah 43:18-21 NAS

SEPTEMBER 3

Not long afterwards He began a tour of the cities and villages of Galilee to announce the coming of the Kingdom of God,

and took His twelve disciples with Him.

Some women went along,

from whom He had cast out demons or whom He had healed;

among them were

Mary Magdalene (Jesus had cast out seven demons from her)

Joanna, Chuza's wife (Chuza was King Herod's business manager and was in charge of his palace and domestic affairs)

Susanna, and many others

who were contributing from their private means to the support of Jesus and His disciples.

Luke 8:1-3 (TLB)

SEPTEMBER 4

PRAYER OF ST. FRANCIS OF ASSISI

A Modern Translation

Lord, make me a channel of thy peace

That where there is hatred,	I may bring love,
That where there is wrong,	I may bring the spirit of forgiveness,
That where there is discord,	I may bring harmony,
That where there is error,	I may bring truth,
That where there is doubt,	I may bring faith,
That where there is despair,	I may bring hope,
That where there are shadows,	I may bring the light,
That where there is sadness,	I may bring joy.

Lord, grant that I may seek rather

To comfort	than to be comforted;
To understand	than to be understood;
To love	than to be loved;

For it is by giving	that one receives;
It is by self-forgetting	that one finds;
It is by forgiving	that one is forgiven;
It is by dying	that one awakens to eternal life.

SEPTEMBER 5

You are my hiding place from every storm of life;
You even keep me from getting into trouble!
You surround me with songs of victory.
I will instruct you (says the Lord) and
guide you along the best pathway for your life;
I will advise you and watch your progress.
Don't be like a senseless horse or mule
that has to have a bit in its mouth to keep it in line!

Psalm 32:7-9 (TLB)

Lord, today I am feeling like this . . .

Stubborn mules go nowhere, fast.

SEPTEMBER 6

For God is greater than man.

Why should you fight against Him just because He does not give account to you of what He does?

For God speaks again and again,

I. In **dreams**, in **visions** of the night when deep sleep falls on men as they lie on their beds.

A. **Opening** their **ears** in times like that,
B. Giving them **wisdom and instruction**,
C. Causing them to **change their minds,**
D. Keeping them from **pride**,
E. Warning them of the **penalties** of sin,
F. Keeping them from **falling** into some trap.

II. Or, God sends **sickness and pain**, even though no bone is broken,

A. So that a man loses all **taste and appetite** for food and doesn't care for even the daintiest dessert.
B. He becomes **thin**, mere skin and bones.
C. Draws near to **death**.

III. But if a **messenger from heaven** (angel) is there

A. To **intercede** for him as a friend
B. To **show him** what is right
    1. Then God pities him and says,
    2. **"Set him free**. Do not make him die, for I have found a substitute."

Then his body will become as healthy as a child's, firm and youthful again.

And when he **prays** to God,

A. **God will hear and answer**.
B. **He will receive** him with **joy**
C. **He will return** him to his duties

And he will declare to his friends

"I sinned, but God let me go. He did not let me die.
I will go on living in the realm of light."

Yes, God often does these things for man - brings back his soul from the pit, so that he may live in the light of the living.

Job 33:12-30 (TLB)

SEPTEMBER 7

After the apostles returned to Jesus
and reported what they had done,

He slipped quietly away with them
toward the city of Bethsaida.

But the crowds found out where He was going,
and followed.

And He welcomed them,
teaching them again about the Kingdom of God

and curing those who were ill.

Luke 9:10-11 (TLB)

SEPTEMBER 8

C O M P A S S I O N

from the Latin words *cum* and *pati*

together meaning to *suffer with*

The original inspiration and compulsion to compile and type this *Caregivers Journal* came in May and June, 1991. It was then laid aside in the demands of caregiving. In September, Ron's behavior became even more highly agitated and confusing. On September 8th I was very upset and desperate for help and insight to know how to help him and to know how to care for him.

"Get out the *Caregivers Journal,*" said the Lord. I did. WOW!! Did I ever need to be freshly reminded about COMPASSION on this day! The original page had the word COMPASSION written the length of the page, and I had drawn hearts for the O's. Thanks! I needed that, Lord!

"Use the Journal daily. I wrote it through you. You typed it. Do you still believe it? Does it really minister and speak to you as a caregiver?"

"OK, Lord. I will use it daily." And I did. From this point on, I have not edited or changed the order of the original writings. They each ministered to me in a very real way on each day that they were typed for, until Ron's death on December 21, 1991.

SEPTEMBER 9

The Spirit of the Lord God is upon me,
Because the Lord has **anointed** me
    To bring **good news to the afflicted**;
    He has sent me to **bind up the brokenhearted**,
    To **proclaim liberty to captives**,
    And **freedom to prisoners;**
    To proclaim the favorable year of the Lord, . . .
    To **comfort all who mourn**, . . .
    Giving them a **garland instead of ashes,**
    The **oil of gladness instead of mourning,**
    The **mantle of praise instead of a spirit of fainting.**
    So they will be called **oaks of righteousness,**
    The planting of the LORD, that **He may be glorified**.

Then they will **rebuild** the ancient ruins,
They will **raise up** the former devastations,
And they will **repair** the ruined cities,
The desolations of many generations.

Instead of your **shame** you will have a **double portion**,
And instead of **humiliation** they will **shout for joy . . .**
    everlasting joy will be theirs. . . .

I will **rejoice** greatly in the LORD,
My soul will exult in my God;
    For He has clothed me with **garments of salvation,**
    He has wrapped me with a **robe of righteousness,**
    As a **bridegroom** decks himself with a garland,
    And as a **bride** adorns herself with her **jewels**.

Isaiah 61:1-4, 7, 10 NAS

THE GRACE OF JESUS CHRIST

191 Jesus Loves Me

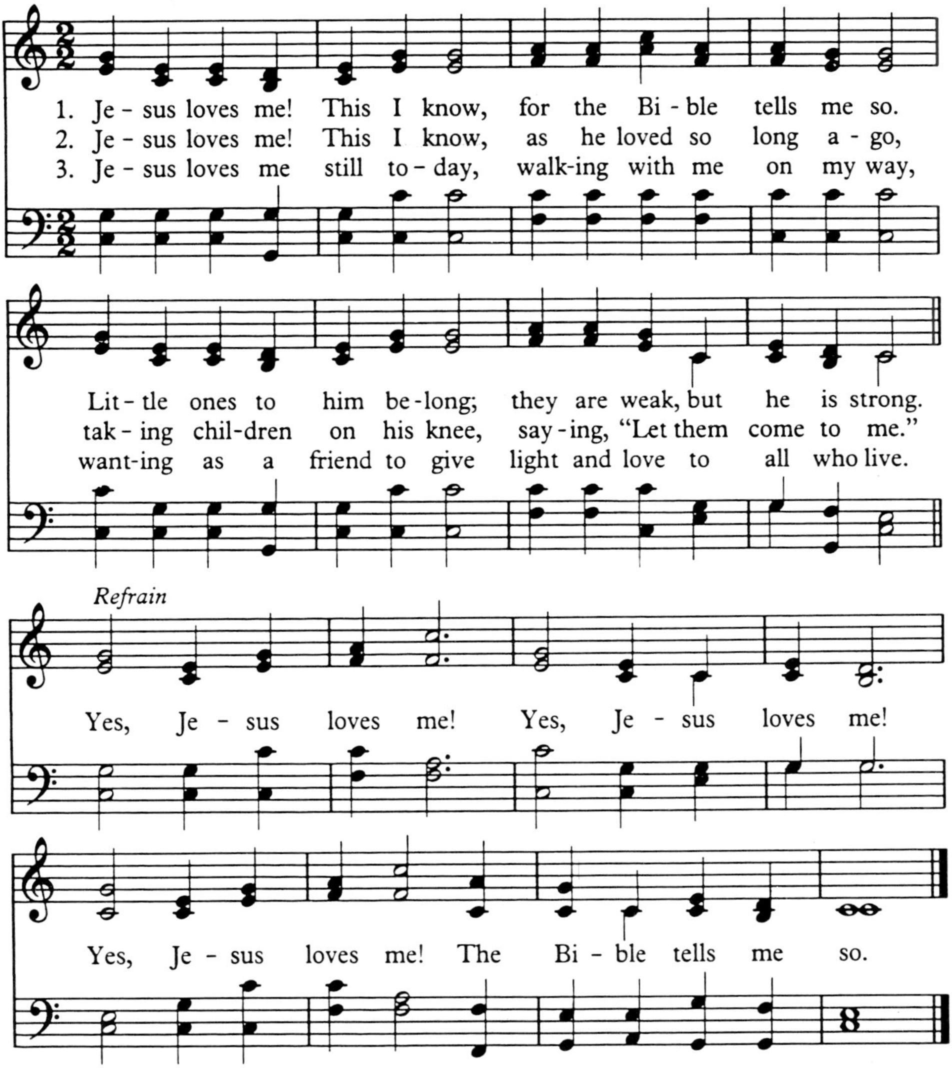
1. Je - sus loves me! This I know, for the Bi - ble tells me so.
2. Je - sus loves me! This I know, as he loved so long a - go,
3. Je - sus loves me still to - day, walk-ing with me on my way,
Lit - tle ones to him be - long; they are weak, but he is strong.
tak - ing chil-dren on his knee, say - ing, "Let them come to me."
want-ing as a friend to give light and love to all who live.
Refrain
Yes, Je - sus loves me! Yes, Je - sus loves me!
Yes, Je - sus loves me! The Bi - ble tells me so.

WORDS: St. 1 Anna B. Warner, 1860; Sts. 2-3 David Rutherford McGuire; trans.:
MUSIC: William B. Bradbury, 1862

JESUS LOVES ME
77.77 with Refrain

SEPTEMBER 11

"Let not your heart be troubled.
You are trusting God, now trust in Me.
There are many homes up there where My Father lives,
And I am going to prepare them for your coming.

When everything is ready,
Then I will come and get you,
so that you can always be ***with me*** *where I am.*

If this weren't so, I would tell you plainly.
And you know where I am going and how to get there."

"No, we don't," Thomas said.
"We haven't any idea where you are going,
so how can we know the way?"

Jesus told him,

"I am the Way - yes, and the Truth and the Life.
No one can get to the Father except by means of Me.
If you had known who I am,
then you would have known who My Father is.
From now on you know Him - and have seen Him!"

John 14:1-7 (TLB)

SEPTEMBER 12

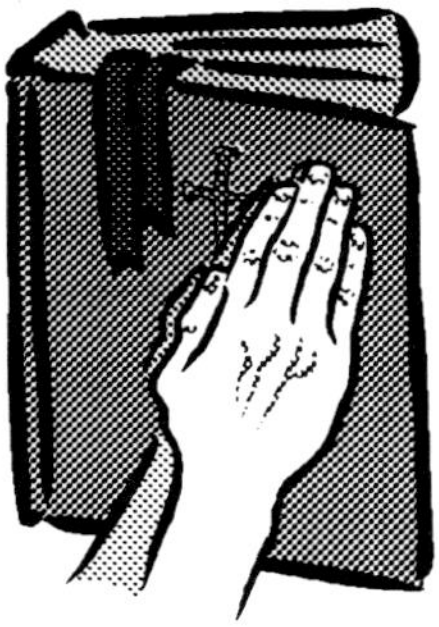

THE DIFFERENCE

I got up early one morning
and rushed right into the day;
I had so much to accomplish
that I didn't have time to pray.

Problems just tumbled about me,
and heavier came each task.
"Why doesn't God help me?" I wondered.
He answered, "You didn't ask."

I wanted to see joy and beauty,
but the day toiled on, gray and bleak,
I wondered why God didn't show me
He said, "But you didn't seek."

I tried to come into God's presence;
I used all my keys at the lock.
God gently and lovingly chided,
"My child, you didn't knock."

I woke up early this morning,
and paused before entering the day;
I had so much to accomplish
that I had to take time to pray.

Alan Grant

SEPTEMBER 13

I **wait** for the LORD,
my soul does **wait**,
And in His **word**
do I **hope**.

Psalm 130:5 NAS

Lord, today I am feeling like this . . .

SEPTEMBER 14

The Lord now chose seventy other disciples and sent them on ahead in pairs to all the towns and villages He planned to visit later.

These were His instructions to them:

1. *"Plead with the Lord of the harvest to send out more laborers to help you, for the harvest is so plentiful and the workers so few.*
2. *Go now, and remember that I am sending you out as lambs among wolves.*
3. *Don't take any money with you, or a beggar's bag, or even an extra pair of shoes.*
4. *And don't waste time along the way.*
5. *Whenever you enter a home, give it your blessing . . .*
6. *When you enter a village, don't shift around from home to home, but stay in one place, eating and drinking without question whatever is set before you.*
7. *And don't hesitate to accept hospitality for the workman is worthy of his wages!*

If a town welcomes you, follow these two rules:

1. *Eat whatever is set before you.*
2. ***Heal the sick**; and as you heal them, say, 'The Kingdom of God is very near you now.' " . . .*

When the seventy disciples returned,
they **joyfully** reported to him,
"Even the demons obey us when we use Your name."

Luke 10:1-9, 17 (TLB)

SEPTEMBER 15

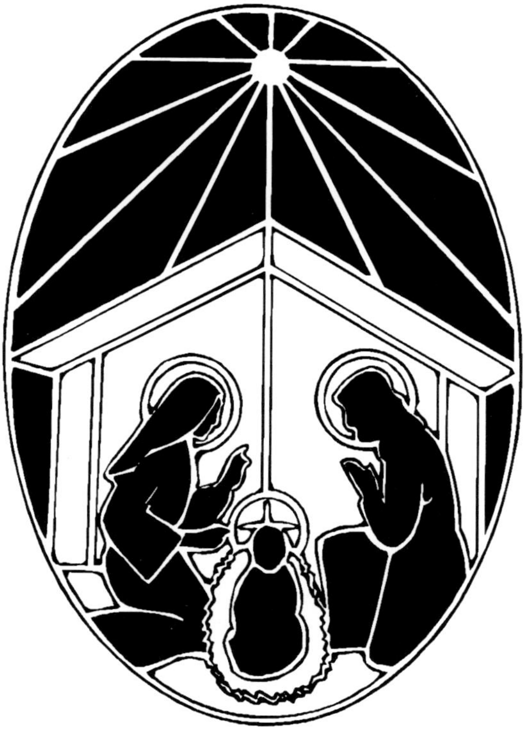

In Him was life,
and the life was the light of men.

And the light shines in the darkness,
and the darkness did not comprehend it.

John 1:4-5 NAS

SEPTEMBER 16

Sing for **joy** to God our **strength**;
Shout joyfully to the God of Jacob.
Raise a song, strike the timbrel,
The sweet sounding lyre with the harp.
Blow the trumpet at the new moon,
At the full moon, on our feast day. . . .

I relieved his shoulder of the **burden**,
His hands were freed from the basket.
You called in trouble, and I rescued you;
I answered you in the hiding place of thunder . . .

I, the LORD, am your God,
Who brought you up from the land of Egypt;
O p e n your mouth **w i d e**
and I will fill it. . . .

But I would feed you with the finest of wheat;
And with honey from the rock,
I would satisfy you.

Psalm 81:1-3, 6-7, 10, 16 NAS

SEPTEMBER 17

JUSTIFYING GRACE

377 It Is Well with My Soul

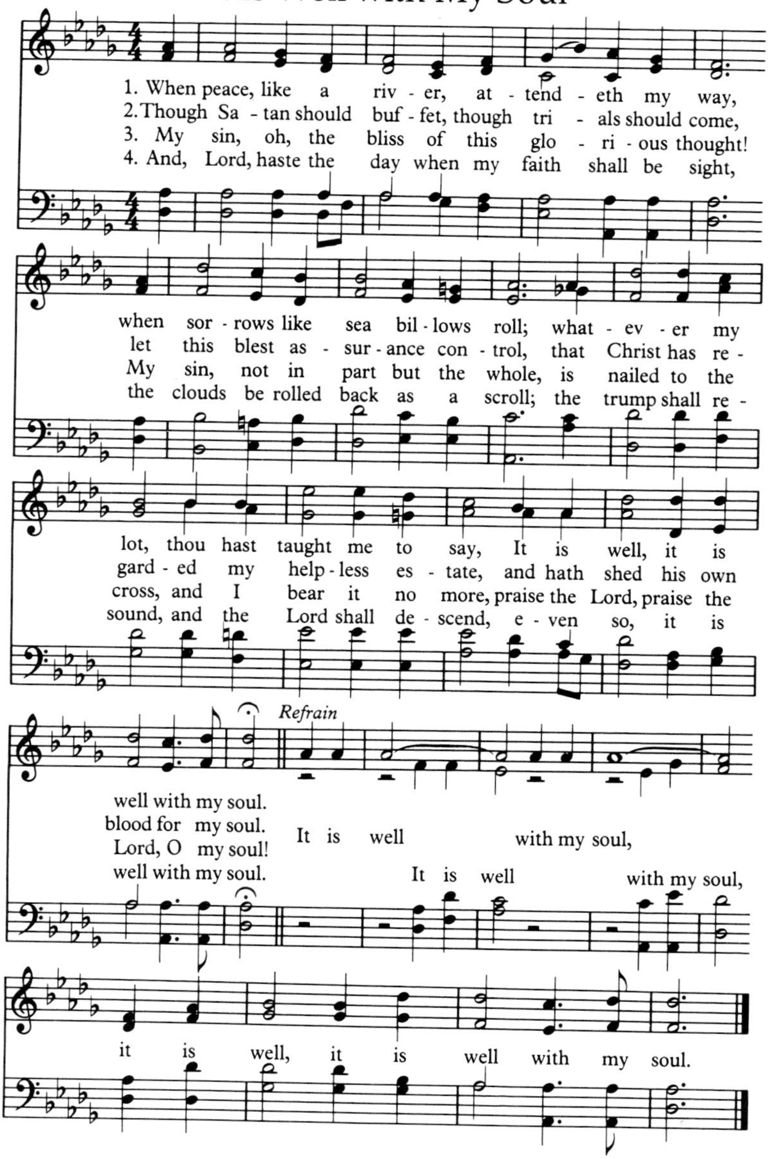

WORDS: Horatio G. Spafford, 1873
MUSIC: Philip P. Bliss, 1876

VILLE DU HAVRE
11 8.11 9 with Refrain

SEPTEMBER 18

Thy **word** is a lamp to my feet,

and a **light** to my path.

Psalm 119:105 NAS

Lord, today I am feeling like this . . .

SEPTEMBER 19

Making the change from a lifetime of employment
to retirement

from a secure small town school
and church-centered lifestyle
to a big city with new friends
to meet and a new church that
worships differently

from an overloaded schedule
to time to make leisurely
activity choices

from serving others
to receiving love from family

from excellent health
to health concerns

I am reminded of the half time of an athletic event.

HALF TIME

The first half was played well
Executed many excellent plays
Scored many points
The first quarter was played with extraordinary
energy and success
The second quarter showed signs of physical exhaustion
No substitutes came in to relieve
Injuries began to occur

Timeouts were called to treat unexpected injuries
or to regroup after receiving a new play from the Coach

Continued on September 20

SEPTEMBER 20

NOW IT IS HALF TIME

Rest . . . . lay on benches and rest
Drink . . . . water to quench thirst
Coach . . . . gives encouragement and instructions
Trainer . . . . works on injuries
Teammates . . . . joke, talk, plan, encourage each other

Second half energy will not be as high
Coach gives new plays that adjust to the game and player situations

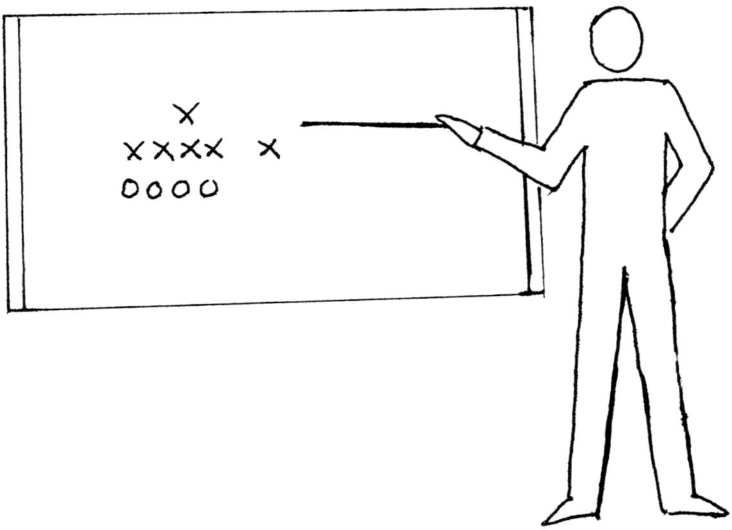

Team returns to the playing field and gets back into the game. There is still time to execute successful plays.

Victory is not claimed or celebrated until the final time has run out.

SEPTEMBER 21

And leaving the multitude,
they took Him along with them,
just as He was, in the **boat**;
and other boats were with Him.

And there arose a **fierce gale of wind,**
and the waves were breaking over the boat
so much that the boat was already filling up.

And He Himself was in the stern,
asleep on the cushion;
and they awoke Him and said to Him,
"Teacher, do you not care that we are perishing?"

And being aroused, He rebuked the wind and said to the sea,
"Hush, be still,"
And the wind died down and
it became perfectly calm.

And He said to them,
"Why are you so timid?
How is it that you have no faith?"
And they became very much afraid and said to one another,
"Who then is this, that even the wind
and the sea obey Him?"

Mark 4:36-41 NAS

Lord, when the **boat of caregiving** that I am in,
fills up with water and I am afraid of drowning,
come and quiet the storm in me and return calm to my life.

SEPTEMBER 22

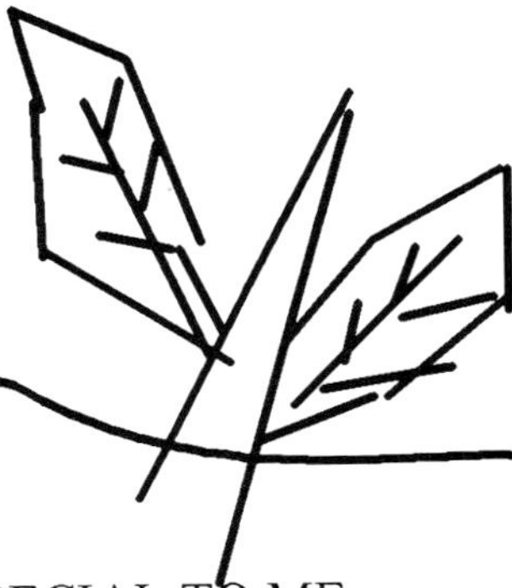

APPLES ARE SPECIAL TO ME
My mother's maiden name was Apple

Apples remind me of the Genesis story of Adam and Eve . . . of the original sin that separated us from God. Genesis 2:15 - 3:22

. . . and apples remind me of the love and forgiveness of the God in three persons . . .

PEEL	protects	GOD THE FATHER
FLESH	goodness	GOD THE SON
CORE	seeds	GOD THE HOLY SPIRIT

Apples raw (new believer)
applesauce (sifted believer)
apple cider (squeezed even more)
apple pie (sweetness of Jesus in me). . .
many ways God can use me.

SEPTEMBER 23

How blessed is he who considers the helpless;
The Lord will deliver him in a day of trouble.

The Lord will protect him,
and keep him alive,
And he shall be called blessed upon the earth;
And do not give him over to the desire of his enemies.

The Lord will sustain him upon his sickbed;
In his illness, Thou dost restore him to health.

Psalm 41:1-3 NAS

SEPTEMBER 24

Jesus, Gentle Shepherd, lead me as a shepherd leads his sheep around danger and to the good pasture.

Lead me through medical decisions, legal situations, daily needs, to the green pasture of Your Peace.

I submit to your shepherding.

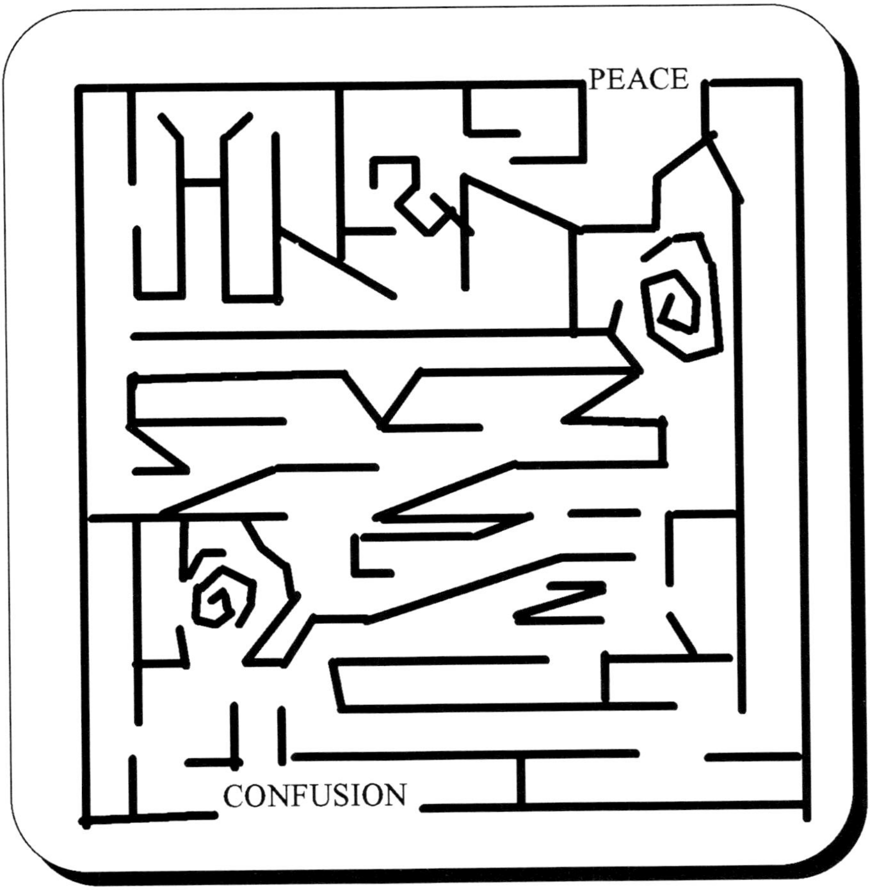

. . . the sheep hear His voice,
and he calls His own sheep by name,
and leads them out.
John 10:3 NAS

SEPTEMBER 25

CAREGIVERS PRAYER

And let us not lose heart in doing good,

for in due time we shall reap

if we do not grow weary.

So then, while we have opportunity,

let us do good to all men,

and especially to those who are of the

household of the faith.

Galatians 6:9-10 NAS

SEPTEMBER 26

THROUGH IT ALL

I've had many tears and sorrows;
I've had questions for tomorrow;
There've been times I didn't know right from wrong;
But in ev'ry situation, God gave blessed consolation,
That my trials come to only make me strong.

Chorus:
THROUGH IT ALL,
THROUGH IT ALL,
Oh! I've learned to trust in Jesus,
I've leaned to trust in God.
THROUGH IT ALL,
THROUGH IT ALL,
Oh! I've learned to depend up on His Word.

I've been to lots of places,
And I've seen a lot of faces;
There've been times I felt so all alone;
But in my lonely hours, yes, those precious lonely hours,
Jesus let me know that I was His own.

I thank God for the mountains,
And I thank Him for the valleys;
I thank Him for the storms He brought me through;
For if I'd never had a problem,
I wouldn't know that He could solve them,
I'd never know what faith in God could do.

Words and Music by Andrae Crouch

SEPTEMBER 27

. . . before they call,
I will answer;
and while they are still speaking,
I will hear.

Isaiah 65:24 NAS

Lord, today I am feeling like this . . .

SEPTEMBER 28

The man wanted to justify (his lack of love for some kinds of people), so he asked,

"Which neighbors?"

Jesus replied with an illustration:

"A Jew going on a trip from Jerusalem to Jericho was attacked by bandits. They stripped him of his clothes and money and beat him up and left him lying half dead beside the road.

By chance a Jewish priest came along;
and when he saw the man lying there,
he crossed to the other side of the road and passed him by.

A Jewish Temple- assistant walked over and
looked at him lying there, but then went on.

But a despised Samaritan came along,
and when he saw him, he felt deep pity.

Kneeling beside him the Samaritan soothed his wounds with medicine and bandaged them.

Then he put the man on his donkey and walked along beside him till they came to an inn, where he nursed him through the night.

The next day he handed the innkeeper two twenty dollar bills and told him to take care of the man. "If his bill runs higher than that," he said, "I'll pay the difference the next time I am here."

Now which of these three would you say was a neighbor to the bandits' victim?"

The man replied, "The one who showed him some pity."

Then Jesus said, *"Yes, now go and do the same."*

Luke 10:29-37 (TLB)

SEPTEMBER 29

For who is our **hope** or **joy** or **crown of exultation?**
Is it not even you, in the presence of our Lord Jesus
at His coming?

1 Thessalonians 2:19 NAS

Blessed is a man who perseveres under trial;
for once he has been approved, he will receive the
crown of life, which the Lord has promised
to those who love Him. James 1:12 NAS

I have fought the good fight,
I have finished the course,
I have kept the faith;
in the future there is laid up for me the
crown of righteousness,
which the Lord, the righteous Judge,
will award to me on that day;
and not only to me but also to all who
have loved His appearing.

2 Timothy 4:7-8 NAS

Everyone who competes in the games
goes into strict training.
They do it to get a crown that will not last;
but we do it to get a **crown** that will last forever.

1 Corinthians 9:25 NIV

SEPTEMBER 30

One thing I have asked from the LORD,
        that I shall seek;
That I may dwell in the house of the LORD
        all the days of my life,
To behold the beauty of the LORD,
        And to meditate in His temple.

For in the day of trouble
        He will conceal me in His tabernacle;
In the secret place of His tent
        He will hide me;
He will lift me up on a rock.

And now my head will be lifted up above
        my enemies around me;
And I will offer in His tent
        sacrifices with **shouts of joy**;
I will sing, yes, I will sing
        praises to the LORD.

Hear, O LORD, when I cry with my voice,
        And be gracious to me and answer me. . . .

I would have despaired unless I had believed that
        I would see the goodness of the LORD
        In the land of the living.

Wait for the LORD;
        Be strong, and let your heart take courage;
                Yes, wait for the LORD.

Psalm 27:4-7, 13-14 NAS

OCTOBER 1

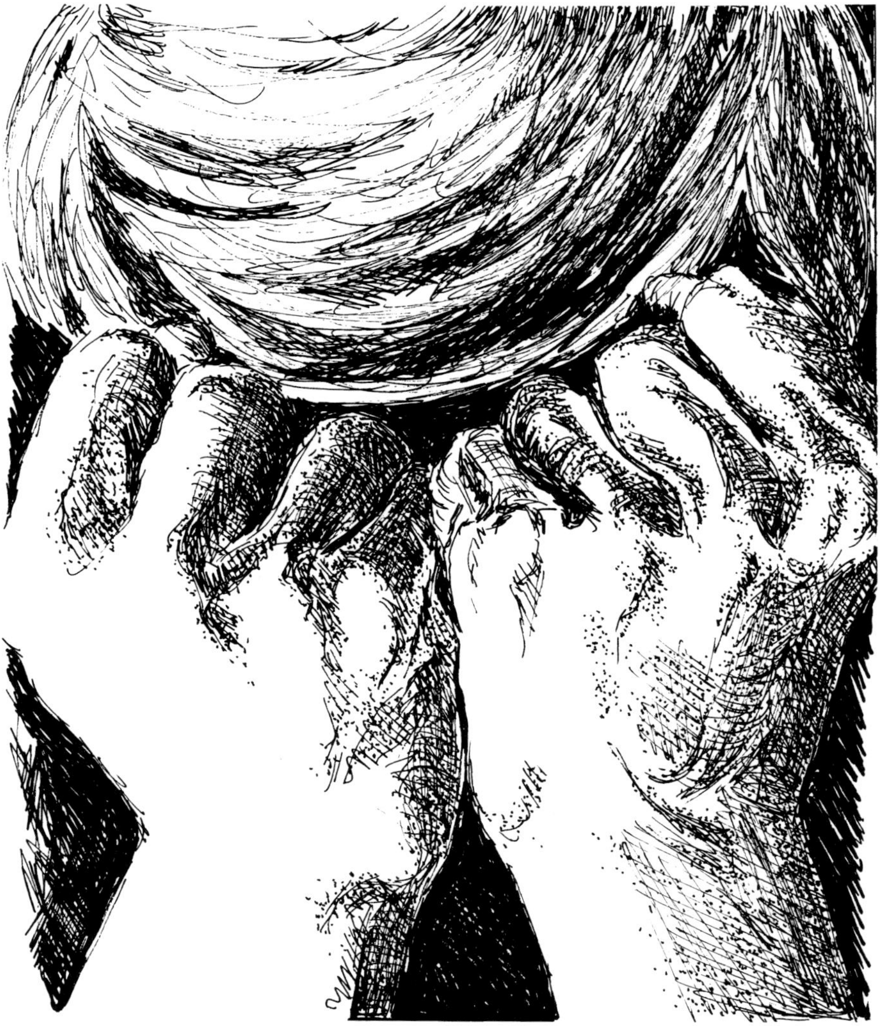

With Clenched Fists

When you are invited to pray, you are asked to open your tightly clenched fists. . . You feel it safer to cling to a sorry past than to trust in a new future. . . . Each time you dare to let go and surrender one of those many fears, your hand opens a little and your palms spread out in a gesture of receiving. You must be patient, of course, very patient until your hands are completely open. . . . you gradually realize that to pray is to live.

With Open Hands by Henri J. M. Nouwen

OCTOBER 2

Simon Peter said to them,
"I am going fishing."

They said to him,
"We will also come with you."

They went out, and got into the boat;
and that night they caught nothing.

But when the day was now breaking,
Jesus stood on the beach;
Yet the disciples did not know that it was Jesus.

Jesus therefore said to them,
"Children, you do not have any fish, do you?"

They answered Him, "No."

And He said to them,
"Cast the net on the right-hand side of the boat,
and you will find a catch."

They cast therefore, and then they were not able to haul it in
because of the great number of fish. . . .

Simon Peter went up, and drew the net to land,
full of large fish, a hundred and fifty-three;
and although there were so many,
the net was not torn.

John 21:3-6, 11 NAS

Lord, Jesus, You are always with me, You know my needs,
You have provided abundantly for my needs,
I want to look to You first and then do the work.

OCTOBER 3

Jesus got up from the supper table,
took off His robe, wrapped a towel around His loins,
poured water into a basin,
and began to wash the disciples' feet
and wipe them with the towel
He had around Him.

After washing their feet
He put on His robe again and sat down and asked,

"Do you understand what I was doing?
You call me 'Master' and 'Lord,'
and you do well to say it, for it is true.
And since I, The Lord and Teacher,
have washed your feet,

you ought to wash each other's feet.

I have given you an example to follow:
do as I have done to you.

How true it is that a servant is not greater than his master.
Nor is the messenger more important than
the one who sends him.
You know these things - now ***do them****!*

This is the path of blessing."

John 13:4-5, 12-17 (TLB)

Master Teacher, I will learn to bless my loved one by
soaking their feet in warm sudsy water,
drying them with a soft fluffy towel, and
massaging each sole with lotion.
Prepare the heart of my loved one to realize my love for them
and my heart to serve them. Prepare their body to relax and
enjoy the touch of my hands.

OCTOBER 4

Your laws are both my **light** and my **counselors**.

Psalm 119:24 (TLB)

Lord, today I am feeling like this . . .

OCTOBER 5

One Sabbath as He was in the home of a member
of the Jewish Council,

> the Pharisees were watching Him like hawks to see if
> He would heal a man who was present
> who was suffering from dropsy.

Jesus said to the Pharisees and legal experts standing around,

> *"Well, is it within the Law to heal a man on the Sabbath day, or not?"*

And when they refused to answer,

> Jesus took the sick man by the hand and healed him
> and sent him away.

Luke 14:1-4 (TLB)

OCTOBER 6

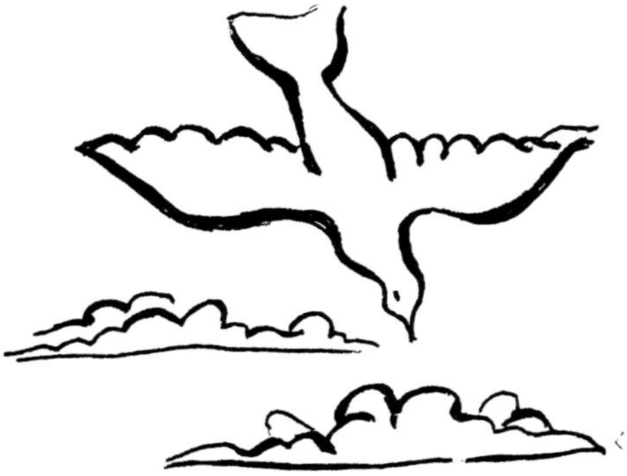

AND THE SPIRIT OF THE LORD
WILL REST ON HIM,

The SPIRIT of WISDOM and UNDERSTANDING,

The SPIRIT of COUNSEL and STRENGTH,

The SPIRIT of KNOWLEDGE and
the FEAR of the LORD

Isaiah 11:2 NAS

OCTOBER 7

Oh, give thanks to the LORD, for He is good;
For His lovingkindness is everlasting.
Let the redeemed of the LORD say so,
Whom He has redeemed from the hand of the adversary,
And gathered from the lands,
From the east and from the west,
From the north and from the south. . . .

Fools, because of their rebellious way,
And because of their iniquities, were afflicted.
Their soul abhorred all kinds of food;
And they drew near to the gates of death.
Then they cried out to the LORD in their trouble;
He saved them out of their distresses.
He sent **His word** and **healed** them,
And delivered them from their destructions.
Let them give thanks to the LORD for His lovingkindness,
And for His wonders to the sons of men!
Let them also offer **sacrifices of thanksgiving**,
And tell of His works with joyful singing. . . .

He changes a wilderness into a pool of water,
And a dry land into springs of water;
And there He makes the hungry to dwell,
So that they may establish an inhabited city,
And sow fields, and plant vineyards,
And gather a fruitful harvest.
Also He blesses them and they multiply greatly;
And He does not let their cattle decrease. . . .

Who is wise?
Let him give heed to these things;

And consider the lovingkindnesses of the LORD.

Psalm 107:1-3, 17-22, 35-38, 43 NAS

OCTOBER 8

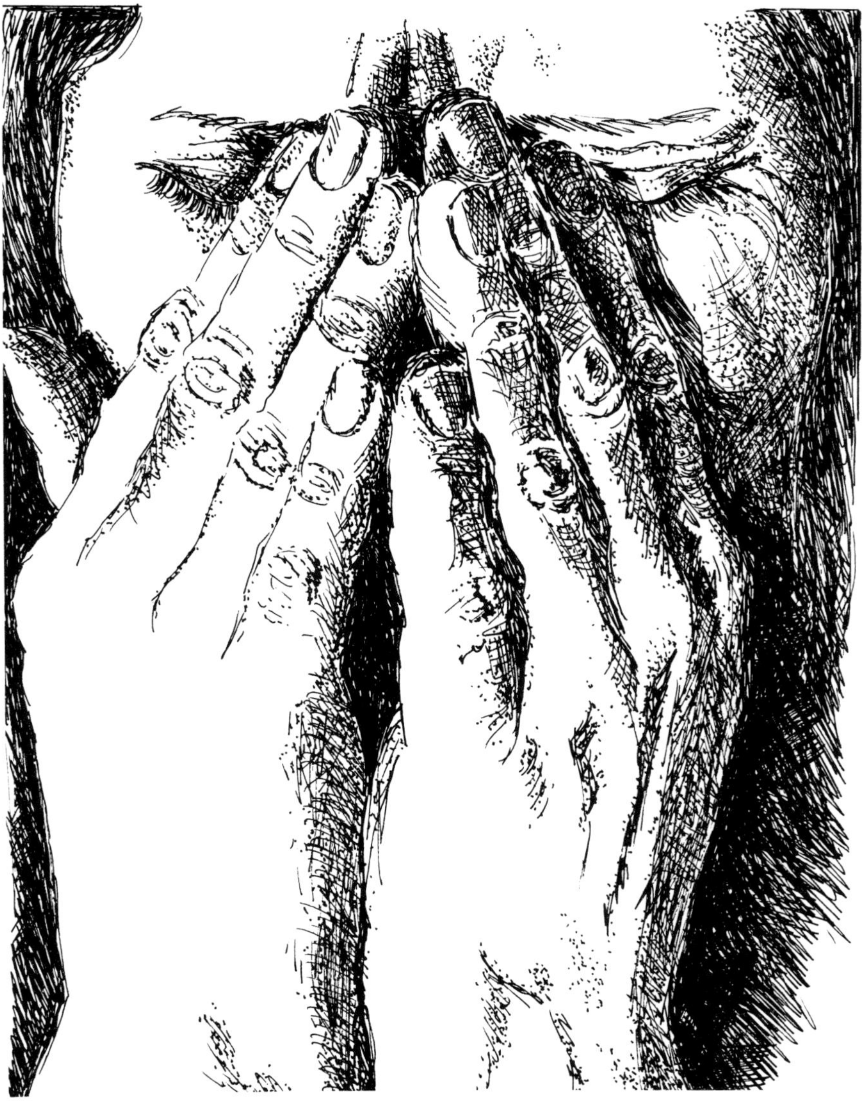

Prayer and Silence

. . . there are two silences: one is frightening, and the other peaceful. . . . But still more difficult than getting rid of these exterior noises is the achievement of inner silence, a silence of the heart.

With Open Hands, Henri J. M. Nouwen

OCTOBER 9

The BE ATTITUDES

One day as the crowds were gathering, He (Jesus) went up the hillside with His disciples and sat down and taught them there.

"Humble men are very fortunate!
for the Kingdom of Heaven is given to them.

Those who mourn are fortunate!
for they shall be comforted.

The meek and lowly are fortunate!
for the whole wide world belongs to them.

HAPPY are those who long to be just and good,
for they shall be completely satisfied.

HAPPY are the kind and merciful,
for they shall be shown mercy.

HAPPY are those whose hearts are pure,
for they shall see God.

HAPPY are those who strive for peace -
they shall be called the sons of God.

HAPPY are those who are persecuted because they are good,
for the Kingdom of Heaven is theirs."

Matthew 5:1-10 (TLB)

OCTOBER 10

Lord, today I am feeling like this . . .

If you get a **lemon,** make **lemonade**.

OCTOBER 11

As they continued onward toward Jerusalem,
they reached the border between Galilee and Samaria,
and as they entered a village there,
ten lepers stood at a distance, crying out,

"Jesus, sir, have mercy on us!"

He looked at them and said,

"Go to the Jewish priest and
show him that you are healed!"

And as they were going,
their leprosy disappeared.

One of them came back to Jesus, shouting,

"Glory to God, "I'm healed!"

He fell flat on the ground in front of Jesus,
face downward in the dust,
thanking Him for what He had done.

This man was a despised Samaritan.

Jesus asked,

"Didn't I heal ten men? Where are the nine?
Does only this foreigner return to give glory to God?"

And Jesus said to the man,

"Stand up and go; your faith has made you well."

Luke 17:11-19 (TLB)

OCTOBER 12

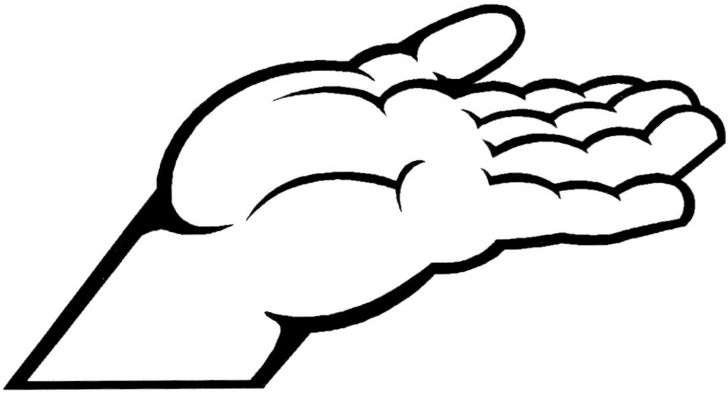

LET

GO

LET

GOD

OCTOBER 13

Blessed be the LORD,
        Because He has heard the voice of my supplication.

The LORD is my strength and my shield;
        My heart trusts in Him,
                and I am helped;
Therefore my heart exults,
        And with my song I shall thank Him.

The LORD is their strength,
        And HE is a saving defense to His anointed.

Save Thy people,
        and bless Thine inheritance;
Be their shepherd also,
        and carry them forever.

Psalm 28:6-9 NAS

OCTOBER 14

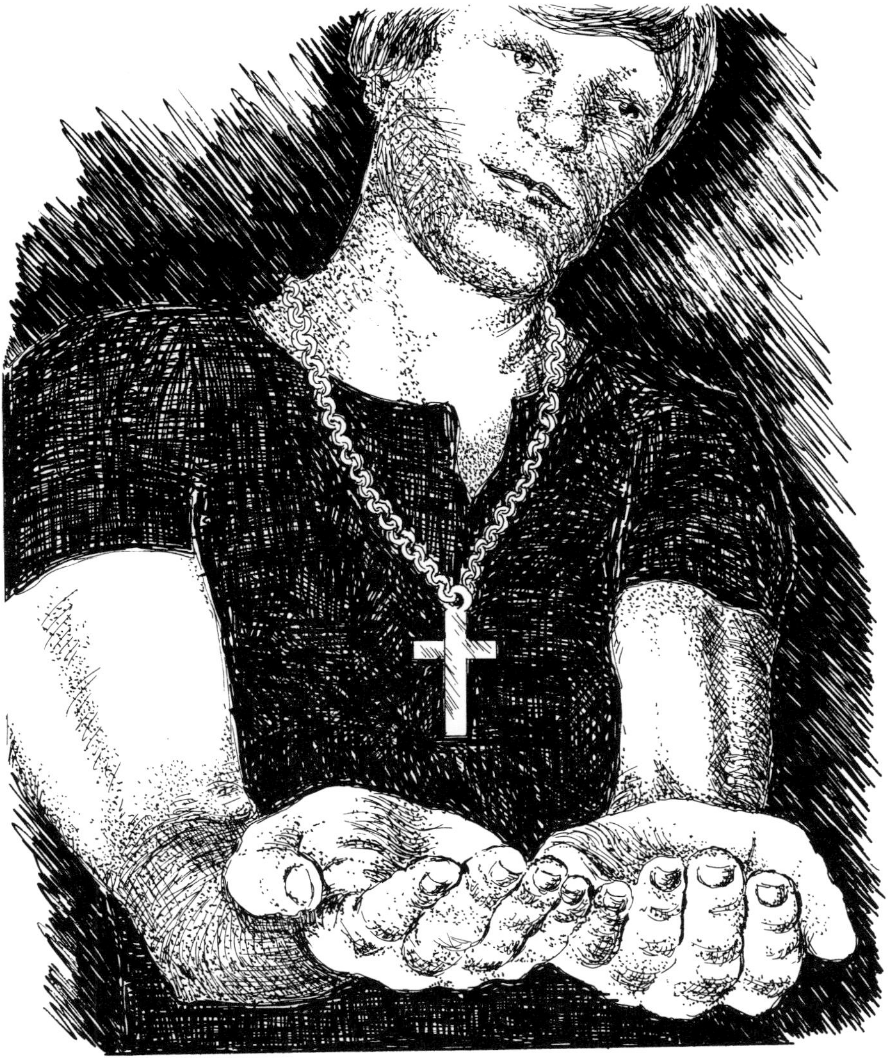

Prayer and Acceptance

Deep silence leads us to realize that prayer is, above all, acceptance. When we pray we are standing with our hands open to the world. . . . Prayer creates that openness in which God is given to us. . . . Prayer gives us the courage to stretch out our arms and to be led.

With Open Hands by Henri J. M. Nouwen

OCTOBER 15

The King of Syria had high admiration for Naaman,
the commander-in-chief of his army,
for he had led his troops to many glorious victories.
So he was a great hero, but he was a **leper**.

Bands of Syrians had invaded the land of Israel and
among their captives was a **little girl** who had been
given to Naaman's wife as a maid.

One day the little girl said to her mistress,
"I wish my master would go to see the prophet in Samaria.
He would heal him of his leprosy!"
Naaman told the king what the little girl had said.

"Go and visit the prophet," the king told him.
"I will send a letter of introduction for you to carry
to the king of Israel."

So Naaman started out, taking gifts of $20,000 in silver,
$60,000 in gold, and ten suits of clothing.

The letter to the king of Israel said:
"The man bringing this letter is my servant Naaman;
I want you to heal him of his leprosy."

When the king of Israel read it, he tore his clothes and said,
"This man sends me a leper to heal!
Am I God, that I can kill and give life?
He is only trying to get an excuse to invade us again."

But when Elisha the prophet heard about the king of Israel's plight,
he sent this message to him:

"Why are you so upset? Send Naaman to me,
and he will learn that there is a true prophet of God
here in Israel."

Continued on October 16

OCTOBER 16

So Naaman arrived with his horses and chariots and
stood at the door of Elisha's home.

> Elisha sent a messenger out to tell him to go and wash in the Jordan River seven times and he would be healed of every trace of his leprosy!
>
> But Naaman was **angry** and **stalked** away.
>
> "Look," he said, "I thought at least he would come out and talk to me! I **expected** him to wave his hand over the leprosy and call upon the name of the Lord his God, and heal me! Aren't the Abana River and Pharpar River of Damascus better than all the rivers of Israel put together? If it's rivers I need, I'll wash at home and get rid of my leprosy."
>
> **So he went away in rage**.

But his officers tried to reason with him and said,

> "If the prophet had told you to do some great thing,
> wouldn't you have done it?
> So you should certainly **obey** him when he says
> simply to go and wash and be cured!"

So Naaman went down to the Jordan River and dipped himself seven times, as the prophet had told him. And his flesh became as healthy as a little child's, **and he was healed**!

Then He and his entire party went back to find the prophet;
they stood **humbly** before him and Naaman said,

> "I know at last that there is no God in all the world
> except in Israel; Now please accept my gifts."

2 Kings 5:1-15 (TLB)

OCTOBER 17

A wise man will hear
and increase in learning,
And a man of understanding
will acquire wise counsel

Proverbs 1:5 NAS

Lord, today I am feeling like this . . .

Lord, lead me to the professional people who can help.

OCTOBER 18

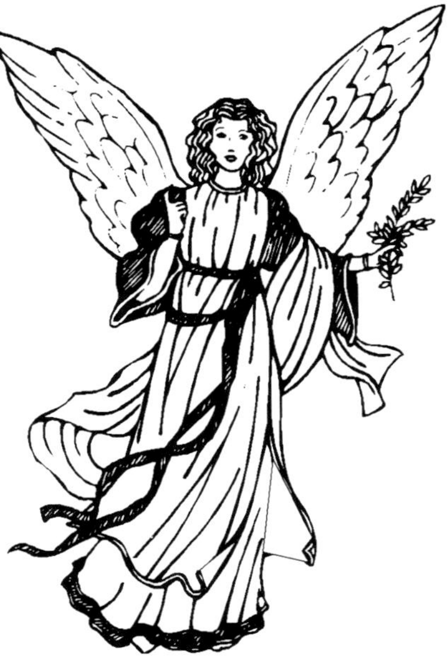

INTERCESSION ANGEL

The angel of the LORD encamps around
those who fear him, and he delivers them.

Psalm 34:7 NIV

STRENGTHENING ANGEL

"Father, if Thou art willing, remove this cup from Me; yet not My will, but Thine be done."
Now an angel from the Heaven appeared to Him strengthening Him.

Luke 22:42-43 NAS

OCTOBER 19

Afterwards Jesus returned to Jerusalem for one of the Jewish religious holidays.

Inside the city, near the Sheep Gate, was Bethesda Pool, with five covered platforms or porches surrounding it.

> Crowds of sick folks - lame, blind, or with paralyzed limbs - lay on the platforms (waiting for a certain movement of the water, for an angel of the Lord came from time to time and disturbed the water, and the first person to step down into it afterwards was healed).

One of the men lying there had been sick for thirty-eight years. When Jesus saw him and knew how long he had been ill, He asked him,

> *"Would you like to get well?"*

"I can't," the sick man said, "for I have no one to help me into the pool at the movement of the water. While I am trying to get there, someone else always gets in ahead of me."

> Jesus told him, *"Stand up, roll up your sleeping mat and go on home!"*

> **Instantly, the man was healed!**
> He rolled up the mat and began walking!

But it was on the Sabbath when this miracle was done.
So the Jewish leaders objected.
They said to the man who was cured,

> "You can't work on the Sabbath!
> It's illegal to carry that sleeping mat!"

Continued on October 20

OCTOBER 20

"The man who healed me told me to," was his reply.

"Who said such a thing as that?" they demanded.

The man didn't know, and Jesus had disappeared into the crowd.
But afterwards Jesus found him in the Temple and told him,

"Now you are well; don't sin as you did before,
or something even worse may happen to you."

Then the man went to find the Jewish leaders and
told them it was Jesus who had healed him.

So they began harassing Jesus as a Sabbath breaker.

But Jesus replied,

"My Father constantly does good,
and I'm following His example."

John 5:1-17 (TLB)

OCTOBER 21

Sing for **joy** in the LORD,
O you righteous ones;
Praise is becoming to the upright. . . .

Sing to Him a new song;
Play skillfully with a **shout of joy.** . . .

The Lord looks from heaven;
He sees all the sons of men; . . .

Behold, the eye of the LORD is on those who fear Him,
On those who hope for His lovingkindness,
To deliver their soul from death,
And to keep them alive in famine.

Our soul **waits** for the LORD;
He is our help and our shield.
For our heart rejoices in Him,
Because we trust in His holy name.

Let Thy lovingkindness, O LORD, be upon us,
According as we have hoped in Thee.

Psalm 33:1, 3, 13, 18-22 NAS

OCTOBER 22

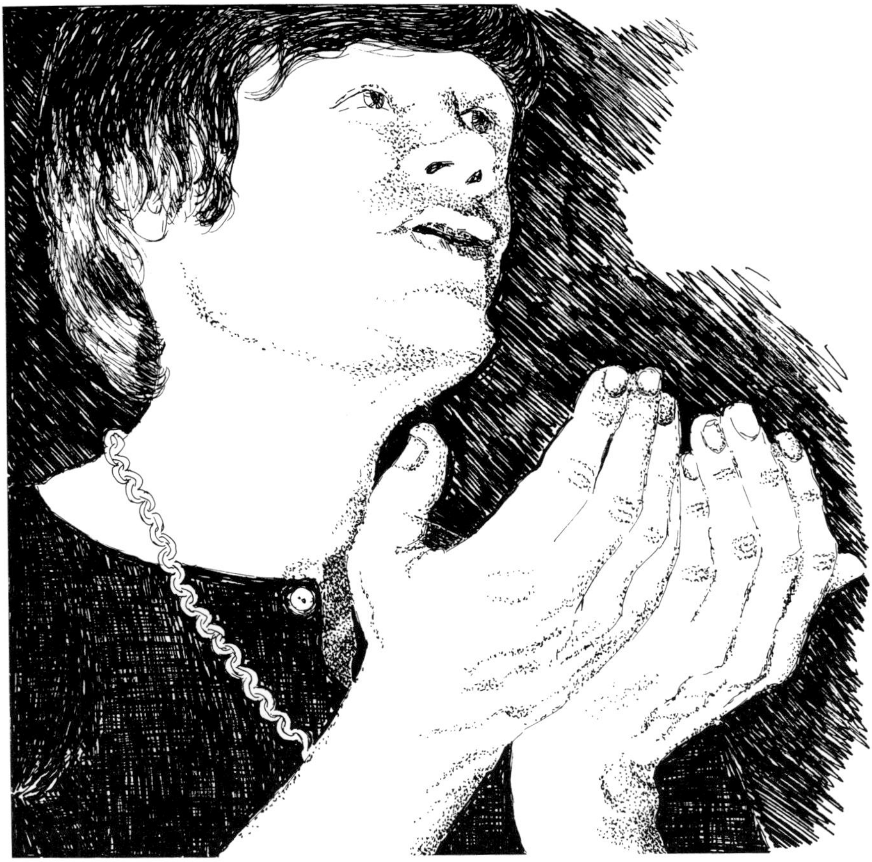

Prayer and Hope

The important thing about prayer is not whether it is classified as petition, thanksgiving or praise, but whether it is a prayer of hope or of little faith. . . . this prayer of little faith carries a great deal of fear and anxiety with it. . . . In the prayer hope, there are no guarantees asked, no conditions posed and no proofs demanded. You expect everything from the other without binding the other in any way. . . . Whenever we pray with hope, we put our lives in the hands of God. Fear and anxiety fade away, and everything we are given and everything we are deprived of is nothing but a finger pointing out the direction of God's hidden promise which one day we shall taste in full.

With Open Hands by Henri J. M. Nouwen

OCTOBER 23

Personalize with your or your loved one's name the

ARMOR OF GOD

Finally, be strong in the Lord, and in the strength of His Might.

Put on the full armor of God, that _______________ may be able to **stand firm** against the schemes of the devil. For your struggle is not against flesh and blood, but against

rulers . . . powers . . . world forces of this darkness,
the spiritual forces of wickedness in the heavenly places.

Therefore, take up the full **armor of God**, that ______________ may be able to resist in the evil day, and having done everything, to stand firm.

STAND FIRM therefore, having

girded your **loins** with **truth, . . .**
put on the **breastplate** of **righteousness, . . .**
shod your **feet** with the preparation of the **gospel of peace; . . .**
taking up the **shield** of **faith**, with which you will be able to extinguish all the flaming missiles of the evil one. . . .
take the **helmet** of **salvation**, . . .
take the **sword** of the **Spirit,** which is the **Word of God**.
with all prayer and petitions **pray at all times in the Spirit**,
and with this in view, be on the alert with all perseverance and petition for **all** the saints,

and **pray** on _______________ behalf that

utterance may be given to ______________ **in the opening of your mouth**, to make known **with boldness** the **mystery** of the **gospel**, for which _______________ is an ambassador in chains; that in proclaiming it _______________ may **speak boldly**, . . .

Ephesians 6:10-20 NAS

OCTOBER 24

Though the fig tree should not blossom,
And there be no fruit on the vines,

Though the yield of the olive should fail,
And the fields produce no food,

Though the flock should be cut off from the fold,
And there be no cattle in the stalls,

Yet I will exult in the Lord,
I will **rejoice** in the God of my salvation.

The Lord God is my strength,
And He has made my feet like hinds' feet,
And makes me walk on my **high places**.

Habakkuk 3:17-19 NAS

OCTOBER 25

Now may the God of **hope**

fill you with all **joy** and **peace** in believing,

that you may abound in **hope**

by the **power** of the **Holy Spirit**.

Romans 15:13 NAS

Lord, today I am feeling like this . . .

OCTOBER 26

As He was walking along, He saw a man blind from birth.

"Master," His disciples asked Him, "why was this man born blind? Was it a result of his own sins or those of his parents?"

"Neither," Jesus answered, *"But to demonstrate the power of God. All of us must quickly carry out the tasks assigned us by the one who sent Me, for there is little time left before the night falls and all work comes to an end. But while I am still here in the world, I give it My light."*

Then He spat on the ground and made mud from the spittle and smoothed the mud over the blind man's eyes, and told him, *"Go and wash in the Pool of Siloam"* (the word "Siloam" means "Sent").

So the man went where he was sent and washed
and **came back seeing!**

His neighbors and others who knew him as a blind beggar asked each other,

"Is this the same fellow - that beggar?"

Some said yes, and some said no.

"It can't be the same, man," they thought,
"but he surely looks like him!"

And the beggar said, "I am the same man!"
Then they asked him how in the world he could see.
What had happened?

And he told them, "A man they call Jesus made mud and smoothed it over my eyes and told me to go to the Pool of Siloam and wash off the mud. I did, and I can see!"

Story continued on October 27 and 28

OCTOBER 27

"Where is He now?" they asked.

"I don't know," he replied.

Then they took the man to the Pharisees. Now as it happened, this all occurred on a Sabbath. Then the Pharisees asked him all about it. So he told them how Jesus had smoothed the mud over his eyes, and when it was washed away, he could see!

Some of them said, "Then this fellow Jesus is not from God, because he is working on the Sabbath."

Others said, "But how could an ordinary sinner do such miracles?" So there was a deep division of opinion among them.

Then the Pharisees turned on the man who had been blind and demanded, "This man who opened your eyes - who do you say he is?"

"I think he must be a prophet sent from God," the man replied.

The Jewish leaders wouldn't believe he had been blind, until they called in his parents and asked them,

"Is this your son? Was he born blind? If so, how can he see?"

His parents replied, "We know this is our son and that he was born blind, but we don't know what happened to make him see, or who did it. He is old enough to speak for himself. Ask him."

They said this in fear of the Jewish leaders who had announced that anyone saying Jesus was the Messiah would be excommunicated.

So for the second time they called in the man who had been blind and told him. "Give the glory to God, not to Jesus, for we know Jesus is an evil person."

"I don't know whether He is good or bad," the man replied, "but I know this:

Continued on October 28

OCTOBER 28

I was blind, and now I see!"

"But what did he do?" they asked. "How did he heal you?"

"**Look**!" the man exclaimed, "I told you once; didn't you listen? Why do you want to hear it again? Do you want to become his disciples too?"

Then they cursed him and said, "You are his disciple, but we are disciples of Moses. We know God has spoken to Moses, but as for this fellow, we don't know anything about him."

"Why, that's very strange!" the man replied. "He can heal blind men, and yet you don't know anything about him! Well, God doesn't listen to evil men, but He has open ears to those who worship Him and do His will. Since the world began there has never been anyone who could open the eyes of someone born blind. If this man were not from God, He couldn't do it."

"You illegitimate bastard, you!" they shouted.
"Are you trying to teach us?" and they threw him out.

When Jesus heard what had happened, He found the man and said,
"Do you believe in the Messiah?"

The man answered, "Who is He, sir, for I want to."

"You have seen Him," Jesus said, *"and He is speaking to you!"*

"Yes, Lord," the man said, "I believe!"

And he **worshiped** Jesus.

Then Jesus told him, "*I have come into the world to give sight to those who are* ***spiritually blind*** *and to show those who think they see that they are blind."*

John 9:1-39 (TLB)

OCTOBER 29

God is our refuge and strength,

A very present help in trouble.

Therefore we will not fear . . .

The LORD of hosts is **with** us . . .

Cease striving (be still) and **know** that **I AM GOD**;

I will be exalted among the nations,

I will be exalted in the earth.

The LORD of hosts is **with** us;

The God of Jacob is our stronghold.

Psalm 46:1-2a, 7a, 10, 11 NAS

OCTOBER 30

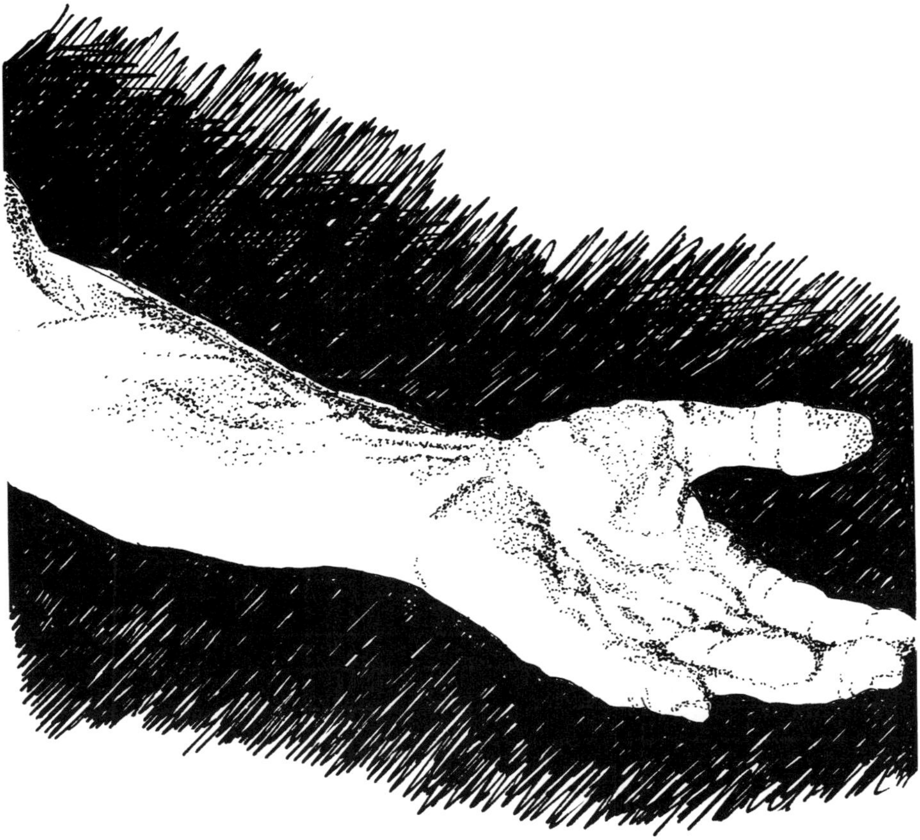

Prayer and Compassion

Prayer has meaning only if it is necessary and indispensable. Prayer is prayer only when we can say that without it, we cannot live. . . . When we pray, we come out of our shelters and not only see our own nakedness but also see that there is no enemy to hide from, only a friend who likes nothing better than to clothe us with a new coat. . . . For compassion means to build a bridge to others without knowing whether they want to be reached. . . . And yet, compassion is possible when it has roots in prayer.

With Open Hands by Henri J. M. Nouwen

OCTOBER 31

REJECTION
Psalm 27:10 NAS

For my father and my mother have forsaken me,
But the Lord will take me up.

REBELLION
Isaiah 53:6 NAS

All of us like sheep have gone astray,
Each of us has turned to his own way . . .

REST
Matthew 11:28 NAS

Come to Me, all who are weary and heavy-laden, and I will give you rest.

REPENTANCE
1 John 1:9 NAS

If we confess our sins, He is faithful and righteous to forgive us our sins and to cleanse us from all unrighteousness.

RESTORATION
Malachi 4:6 NAS

. . . restore the hearts of the Fathers to their children
and the hearts of the children to their Fathers . . .

REBUILD
Haggai 1:8 NAS

"Go up to the mountains,
bring wood and
rebuild the temple,
that I may be pleased with it
and be glorified,"
says the Lord.

NOVEMBER 1

. . . since we have so great a cloud of witnesses surrounding us,
let us also lay aside every encumbrance,
and the sin which so easily entangles us,
and let us run with endurance the race that is set before us.

Hebrews 12:1 NAS

Lord, today I am feeling like this . . .

NOVEMBER 2

But even as He said this, a mob approached, led by Judas, one of His twelve disciples.

Judas walked over to Jesus and kissed Him on the cheek in friendly greeting.

But Jesus said, *"Judas, how can you do this - betray the Messiah with a kiss?"*

When the other disciples saw what was about to happen, they exclaimed, "Master, shall we fight? We brought along the swords!"

And one of them slashed at the High Priest's servant, and cut off his right ear.

But Jesus said, *"Don't resist any more."*

And He touched the place where the man's ear had been and restored it.

Luke 22:47-51 (TLB)

NOVEMBER 3

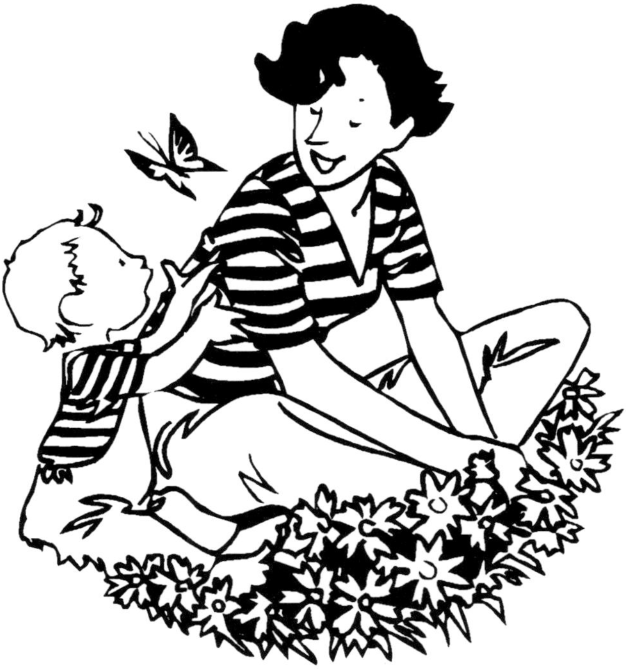

If my thoughts and prayers were butterflies,
every time I set them free they would fly to you,
surrounding you with joy and beauty to brighten your day.

NOVEMBER 4

Then Goliath, a Philistine champion from Gath, came out of the Philistine ranks to face the forces of Israel. He was a giant of a man, measuring **over nine feet tall**! He wore a bronze helmet, a two-hundred pound coat of mail, bronze leggings, and carried a bronze javelin several inches thick, tipped with a twenty-five pound iron spearhead, and his armor bearer walked ahead of him with a huge shield. . . .

As soon as they saw him (Goliath) the Israeli army began to run away in fright.

"Don't worry about a thing," David told him (King Saul). "I'll take care of this Philistine!"

"Don't be ridiculous!" Saul replied. "How can a kid like you fight with a man like him? You are only a boy and he has been in the army since he was a boy!"

But David persisted. "The Lord who saved me from the claws and teeth of the lion and the bear will save me from this Philistine!"

Saul finally consented, "All right, go ahead," he said, "and may the Lord be with you!"

David shouted in reply (to Goliath), "You come to me with a sword and a spear, but I come to you in the name of the Lord of the armies of heaven and of Israel - the very God whom you have defied."

So David conquered the Philistine giant with a sling and a stone.

Selected verses from 1 Samuel 17 (TLB)

Lord, help me to remember that the battle is Yours and that You will give the victory. Open my eyes to see the "stones and sling" You have given me. Fill me with courage to pick them up and use them.

NOVEMBER 5

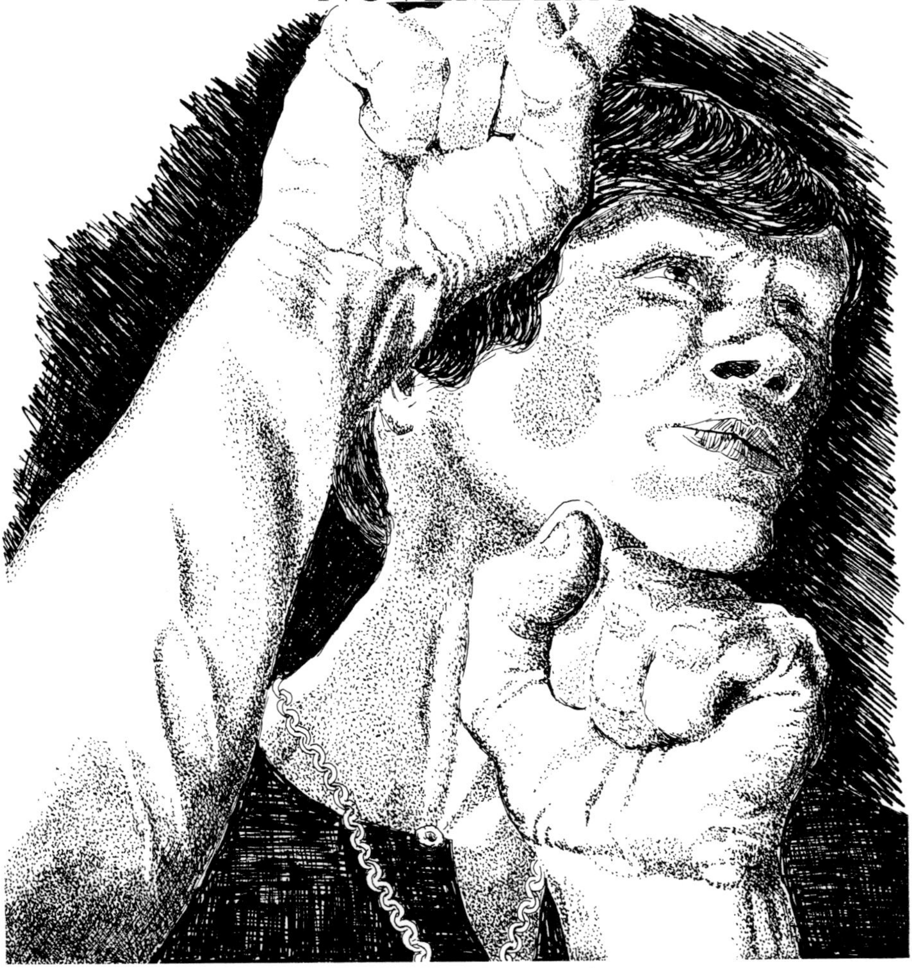

Prayer and Revolution

As your life becomes more and more a prayer, you not only come to a deeper insight into yourself and your neighbor, but you also develop a better feeling for the pulse of the world you live in. If you are really praying, you can't help but have critical questions about the great problems with which the world is grappling, and you can't avoid the thought that a conversion is not only necessary for yourself and your neighbor, but for the entire human community. The conversion of the world calls for a prophetic witness who dares to criticize the world.

With Open Hands by Henri J. M. Nouwen

NOVEMBER 6

You have seen me tossing and turning through the night.
You have collected all my **tears** and
preserved them in **Your bottle!**

Psalms 56:8 (TLB)

Six stone waterpots were standing there; . . . and held perhaps
twenty to thirty gallons each.
Then Jesus told the servants to fill them to the brim with **water**.
When this was done He said,
"Dip some out and take it to the master of ceremonies."

When the master of ceremonies tasted the **water** that was now **wine**, not knowing where it had come from (though, of course, the servants did), he called the bridegroom over.

"This is wonderful stuff!" He said.
"You're different from most. Usually a host uses the best wine first, and afterwards, when everyone is full and doesn't care, then he brings out the less expensive brands."

But you have kept the best for last!"

John 2:6-10 (TLB)

Jesus, the Bridegroom, I have cried gallons of tears. You have collected them all. And now You have turned them into Your wine of joy!!!
I am drunk on Your Spirit. You are making my last mature years the very best part of my life. I celebrate the joy of the wedding of my heart with yours!!! May I serve this new wine You have given me to my loved ones and to others who are ready to receive Your Living Water.

NOVEMBER 7

PAIN HURTS

The human body is not so defenseless that it merely shouts a warning, swells red with injury, and abandons the struggle. If I had to summarize the grand design of pain in one phrase it would be this: pain is directional. It hurts not in order to cause discomfort, but to demand a change in response to danger. And hypersensitivity occurs not as part of a cruel scheme to introduce even more suffering into the body, but as a quick adaptation to force the rest of the body to devote more attention to the vulnerable part. . . .

Sufferers of chronic pain care only about how to turn it off. . . . Pain is no longer a directional signal that points to something else; it is a demon that dominates and immobilizes. . . . Pain management . . teaches patients to live comfortably despite the disease. . . .

We who are strong help the weak. But in handling chronic, long-term pain, the church still seems in its infancy. . . .

Intense suffering provokes a sudden outpouring of aid, but people soon tire of hearing about depressing conditions. . . . No longer a motivator and stimulus for action, the pain becomes a dull, ineffective throb. It has worn us down. . . .

People with chronic pain, such as quadriplegics or the parents of retarded children, describe a common pattern: friends and church members respond initially with sympathy and compassion, but over time they lose interest. Most people find an ordeal with no end in sight unsettling, and can even come to resent the person who is suffering. . . .

A body's health can be measured in large part by its instinctive reaction to nagging, chronic pain. Management of pain requires a delicate balance between proper sensitivity, to determine its cause and mobilize a response, and enough inner strength to keep the pain from dominating the whole person.

NOVEMBER 8

. . . Jesus knelt down and began to pray, saying,

"Father, if Thou art willing, remove this cup from Me;
yet not My will, but Thine be done."

Now an **angel** from heaven appeared to Him, **strengthening** Him.
Luke 22:41-43 NAS

Lord, today I am feeling like this . . .

God didn't say it would be easy . . .
. . . He just said **"Do it!"**

NOVEMBER 9

Peter and John went to the Temple one afternoon to take part in the three o'clock daily prayer meeting.

As they approached the Temple, they saw a man lame
from birth carried along the street and laid beside the
Temple gate - the one called The Beautiful Gate -
as was his custom every day.

As Peter and John were passing by,
he asked them for some money.

They looked at him intently, and then Peter said,

"Look here!"

The lame man looked at them eagerly, expecting a gift.

But Peter said,

"We don't have any money for you! But I'll give you something else! I command you in the name of Jesus Christ of Nazareth, **walk**!"

Then Peter took the lame man by the hand and pulled him to his feet. And as he did, the man's feet and ankle-bones were healed and strengthened so that he came up with a leap, stood there a moment and began walking!

Then **walking,**
leaping,
and praising God,

he went into the Temple with them.

Acts 3:1-8 (TLB)

NOVEMBER 10

The righteous man perishes,
and no man takes it to heart;
And devout men are taken away,
while no one understands.
For the righteous man is taken away from evil,

He enters into peace;
They rest in their beds,
Each one who walked in his upright way.

Isaiah 57:1,2 NAS

NOVEMBER 11

MY SON/MY DAUGHTER

WISDOM	WHY
Do Not Forget My Teaching, but let your heart keep my commandments;	1. For length of days 2. Years of life 3. Peace they will add to you
Do Not Let Kindness and Truth Leave You; Bind them around your neck, Write them on the tablet of your heart	1. So you will find favor and good repute in the sight of God and man.
Trust in the Lord With All Your Heart, and do not lean on your own understanding. In all your ways acknowledge Him,	1. And He will make your paths straight.
Do Not Be Wise in Your Own Eyes Fear the Lordand turn away from evil.	1. It will be healing to your body, 2. Refreshment to your bones.
Honor the Lord From Your Wealth, And from the first of all your produce;	1. So your barns will be filled with plenty, 2. And your vats will overflow with new wine.
Do Not Reject the Discipline Of the Lord, or loathe His reproof,	1. For whom the Lord loves He reproves, 2. Even as a father, the son in whom He delights.

Proverbs 3:1-12 NAS

NOVEMBER 12

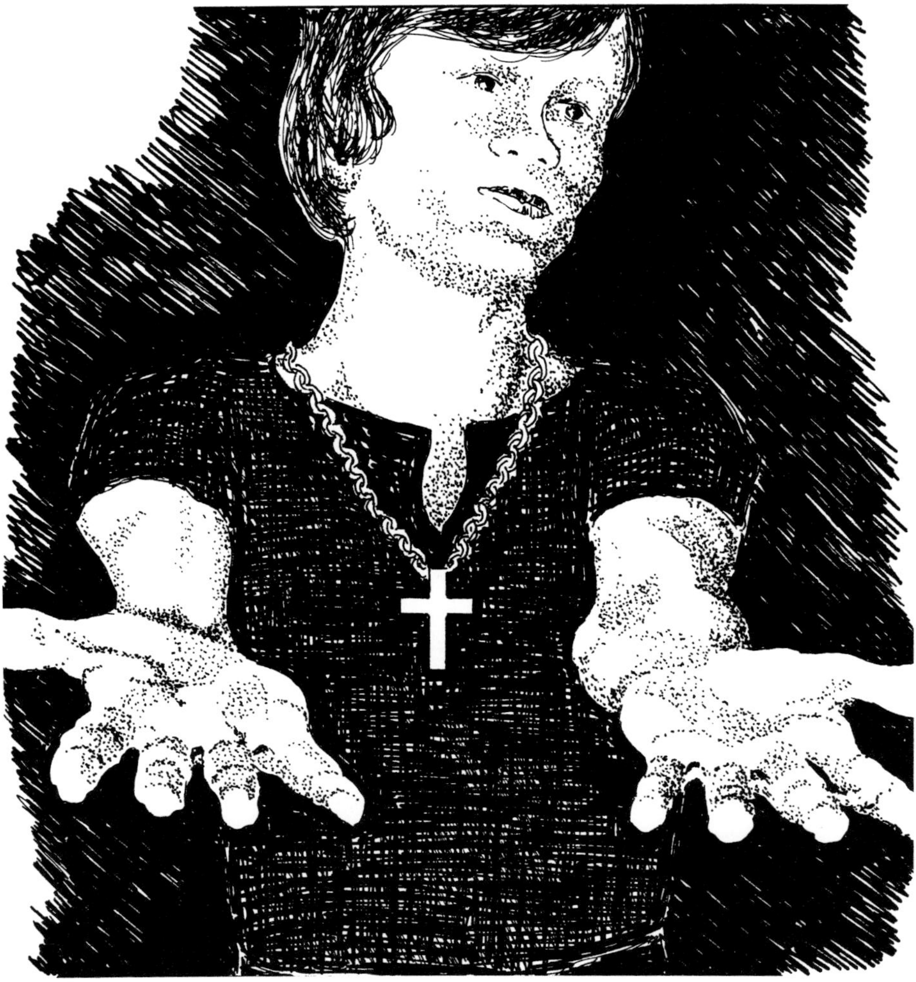

With Open Hands

To pray means to open your hands before God. It means slowly relaxing the tension which squeezes your hands together and accepting your existence with an increasing readiness, not as a possession to defend, but as a gift to receive. . . . In the end, a life of prayer is a life with open hands where we are not ashamed of our weakness but realize that it is more perfect for us to be led by the Other than to try to hold everything in our own hands.

With Open Hands by Henri J. M. Nouwen

NOVEMBER 13

For day by day
men came to David to **help him**,
until there was a great army
like the army of God.
1 Chronicles 12:22 NAS

Lord, today I am feeling like this . . .

NOVEMBER 14

Personalize with your or your loved one's name

SUFFERING = COMFORT

Blessed be the God and Father of our Lord Jesus Christ,
the Father of mercies and God of all comfort;
who comforts ____________ in all ____________affliction
so that ____________ may be able to comfort those
who are in any affliction with the comfort
with which ____________ is comforted by God.
For just as the sufferings of Christ are ____________ in abundance,
so also ____________ comfort is abundant through Christ.
But if ____________ is afflicted,
it is for your comfort and salvation;
or if ____________is comforted,
it is for your comfort
which is effective in the patient enduring of the
same sufferings which we also suffer;
And our hope for ____________ is firmly grounded,
knowing that as ____________ is a sharer of our sufferings,
so also ____________ is a sharer of our comfort.
For we do not want ____________ to be unaware, brethren,
of our affliction which came to us in Asia,
that we were burdened excessively,
beyond our strength,
so that we despaired even of life;
indeed, we had the sentence of death within ourselves
in order that we should not trust in ourselves,
but in God who raises the dead;
who delivered us from so great a peril of death,
and will deliver us, He on whom we have set our hope.

And He will yet deliver ____________

____________also joining in helping us through ____________ prayers,
that thanks may be given by many persons on __________behalf
for the favor bestowed upon ______ through the prayers of many.

2 Corinthians 1:3-11 NAS

NOVEMBER 15

Be **strong** and **courageous, do not fear or be dismayed . . .**

for the one with us is greater than the one with him.

2 Chronicles 32:7 NAS

Lord, today I am feeling like this . . .

NOVEMBER 16

Now when Job's three friends heard of all this adversity
that had come upon him,

they came each one from his own place,

Eliphaz the Temanite,
Bildad the Shuhite, and
Zophar the Naamathite; and

they made an appointment together to come
to sympathize with him and comfort him.

And when they lifted up their eyes at a distance,
and did not recognize him,
they raised their voices and wept.
And each of them tore his robe,
and they threw dust over their heads toward the sky.

Then they sat down on the ground with him
for seven days and seven nights
with no one speaking a word to him,
for they saw that his pain was very great.

Job 2:11-13 NAS

God of Comfort, thank you for the friends who know how to be a comfort to me just by their presence.

NOVEMBER 17

Jesus said,

"Come to Me, all who are weary and heavy-laden,
and I will give you rest.

Take My yoke upon you, and learn from Me,
for I am gentle and humble in heart;
and you shall find rest for your souls.

For My yoke is easy,
and My load is light."

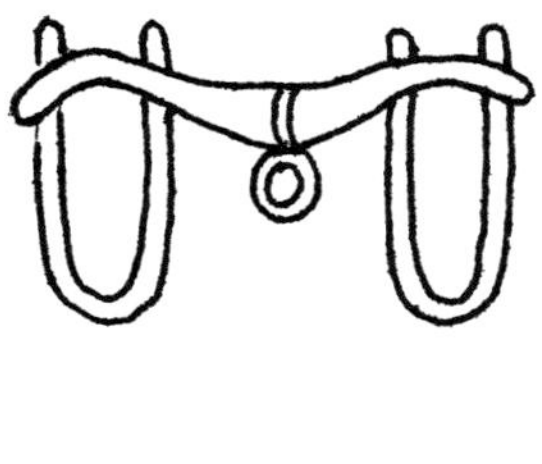

Matthew 11:28-30 NAS

NOVEMBER 18

LORD, BE WITH US IN
THE SEASONS OF OUR LIFE

Spring
Childhood
New Growth
Joy, Laughter

Summer
Youth
Growing
Courage

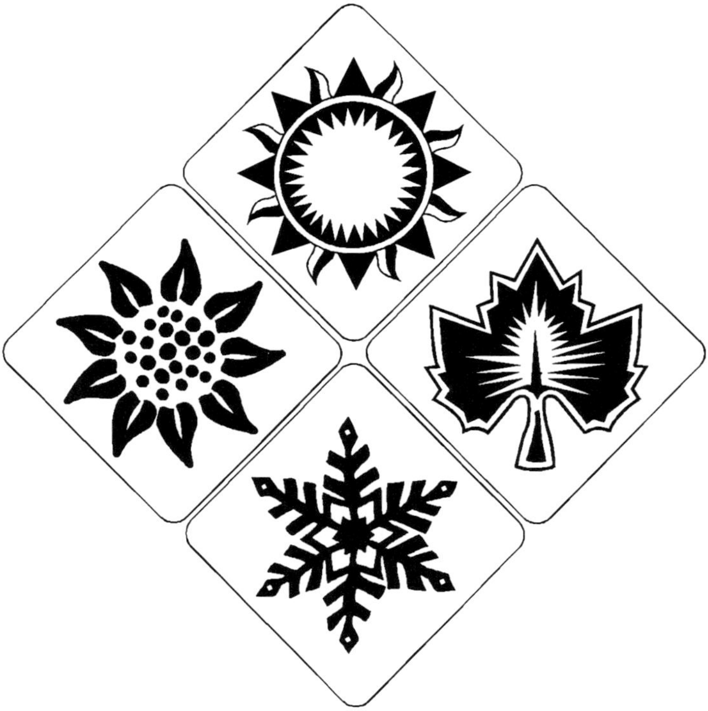

Fall
Adulthood
Productive
Giving

Winter
Old Age
Calm, Rest
Wisdom

NOVEMBER 19

You made all the delicate, inner parts of my body,
and knit them together in my mother's womb.

Thank you for making me so wonderfully complex!
It is amazing to think about.
Your workmanship is marvelous -
and how well I know it.

You were there while I was being formed in utter seclusion!
You saw me before I was born and
scheduled each day of my life before I began to breathe.

Every day was recorded in your Book!

How precious it is, Lord, to realize that you are
thinking about me constantly!
I can't even count how many times a day
your thoughts turn towards me.
And when I waken in the morning,
you are still thinking of me! . . .

Search me, O God, and know my heart;
test my thoughts.
Point out anything you find in me that makes you sad,
and lead me along the path of everlasting life.

Psalms 139:13-18, 23-24 (TLB)

NOVEMBER 20

I love the LORD,
for he heard my voice; he heard my cry for mercy.
Because he turned his ear to me,
I will call on him as long as I live.

The cords of death entangled me,
the anguish of the grave came upon me;
I was overcome by trouble and sorrow.

Then I called on the name of the LORD:
"O LORD, SAVE ME!"

The LORD is gracious and righteous,
our God is full of compassion.
The LORD protects the simplehearted;
when I was in great need, he saved me.
Be at rest once more, O my soul,
for the LORD has been good to you.

For you, O LORD, have delivered my soul from death,
my eyes from tears,
my feet from stumbling,
that I may walk before the LORD in the land of the living.
I believed; therefore I said,
"I am greatly afflicted."
And in my dismay I said,
"All men are liars."

How can I repay the LORD for all his goodness to me?
I will lift up the cup of salvation
and call on the name of the LORD.
I will fulfill my vows to the LORD
in the presence of all his people.

Precious in the sight of the LORD
is the death of his saints.

Psalm 116:1-15 NIV

NOVEMBER 21

Moses therefore said to them,
"Wait, and I will listen to what the Lord
will command concerning you."

Numbers 9:8 NAS

Lord, today I am feeling like this . . .

Wait for godly counselors to help me see God's viewpoint.

NOVEMBER 22

While they were talking to the people, the chief priests, the captain of the Temple police, and some of the Sadducees came over to them, very disturbed that Peter and John were claiming that Jesus had risen from the dead.

> They arrested them and since it was already evening, jailed them overnight.

But many of the people who heard their message believed it, so that the number of believers now reached a new high of about 5,000 men!

> The next day it happened that the Council of all the Jewish leaders was in session in Jerusalem - Annas the High Priest was there, and Caiaphas, John, Alexander, and others of the High Priest's relatives.

So the two disciples were brought in before them.

> "By what power, or by whose authority have you done this?" the Council demanded.

Then Peter, **filled with the Holy Spirit,** said to them,

"Honorable leaders and elders of our nation, if you mean the good deed done to the cripple, and how **he was healed**, let me clearly state to you and to all the people of Israel that it was **done in the name and power of Jesus from Nazareth, the Messiah,** the man you crucified - but God raised back to life again. It is by his authority that this man stands here healed! For Jesus the Messiah is (the one referred to in the Scriptures when they speak of) a 'stone discarded by the builders which became the capstone of the arch.' There is salvation in no one else! Under all heaven there is no other name for men to call upon to save them."

Continued on November 23

NOVEMBER 23

When the Council saw the boldness of Peter and John, and could see that they were obviously uneducated non-professionals, they were amazed and realized what being with Jesus had done for them!

> And the Council could hardly discredit the healing when the man they had healed was standing right there beside them!

So they sent them out of the Council chamber and conferred among themselves.

"What shall we do with these men?" they asked each other. "We can't deny that they have done a tremendous miracle, and everybody in Jerusalem knows about it. But perhaps we can stop them from spreading their propaganda. We'll tell them that if they do it again we'll really throw the book at them." So they called them back in, and told them never again to speak about Jesus.

> But Peter and John replied. "You decide whether God wants us to obey you instead of him! We cannot stop telling about the wonderful things we saw Jesus do and heard him say."

The Council then threatened them further, and finally let them go because they didn't know how to punish them without starting a riot. For everyone was praising God for this wonderful miracle - the healing of a man who had been lame for forty years.

As soon as they were freed, Peter and John found the other disciples and told them what the Council had said.

Then all the believers untied in this prayer:

See Acts 4:24-30 for the prayer.

Acts 4:1-24 (TLB)

NOVEMBER 24

And they (mothers) were bringing children to Him
so that He might **touch** them.

And the disciples rebuked them.

But when Jesus saw this, He was indignant and said to them,

"Permit the children to come to Me; do not hinder them;
for the kingdom of God belongs to such as these.
Truly I say to you, whoever does not receive the kingdom of God
like a child shall not enter it at all."

And He took them in His arms and began **blessing** them,
laying His hands upon them. (Gentle Touch)

Mark 10:13-16 NAS

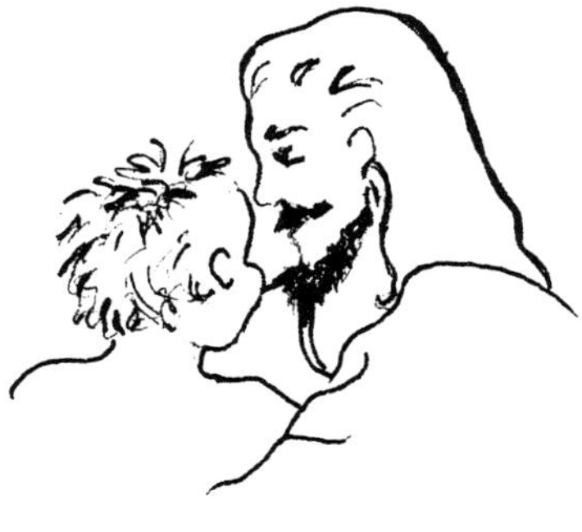

Gentle Jesus, help me to realize that the **touches** You give and the **words** You speak are gentle and tender and loving. Erase the ugly touches and words that have been given to me by the humans in my life. Replace those memories with your loving words and touches. Open my ears to hear Your words of **blessing** spoken to me.

NOVEMBER 25

GOD IS ABLE

GOD IS ABLE to make it up to you
by giving you everything you need and more,
so that there will not only be enough for your own needs
but plenty left over to give joyfully to others.
2 Corinthians 9:8 (TLB)

He (Abraham) considered that **GOD IS ABLE**
to raise men even from the dead . . .
Hebrews 11:19 NAS

If we are thrown into the flaming furnace,
our **GOD IS ABLE** to deliver us;
and He will deliver us out of your hand . . .
Daniel 3:17 (TLB)

And after He (Jesus) had come into the house,
the blind men came up to Him, and Jesus said to them,
*"Do you believe that **I AM ABLE** to do this?"*
They said to Him, " Yes, Lord."
Matthew 9:28 NAS

Now glory be to **God** who by His mighty **power**
at work **within us IS ABLE** to do far more than
we would ever dare to ask or even dream of -
infinitely beyond our highest
prayers desires
thoughts hopes
Ephesians 3:20 (TLB)

That is why I (Paul) am suffering here in jail
and I am certainly not ashamed of it,
for I know the one in whom I trust, and I am sure that **HE IS ABLE**
to safely guard all that I have given him until the day of His return.
2 Timothy 1:12 (TLB)

NOVEMBER 26

O Lord, you alone are my hope;
I've trusted you from childhood.
Yes, you have been with me from birth
and have helped me constantly -
no wonder I am always praising you!
My success - at which so many stand amazed -
is because you are my mighty protector.
All day long I'll praise and honor you, O God,
for all that you have done for me.
And now, in my old age, don't set me aside.
Don't forsake me now when my strength is failing.
My enemies are whispering,
"God has forsaken him! Now we can get him.
There is no one to help him now!"
O God, don't stay away ! Come quickly!
Help! Destroy them!
Cover them with failure and disgrace -
these enemies of mine.
I will keep on expecting you to help me.
I praise you more and more.
I cannot count the times when you have faithfully rescued me from danger. I will tell everyone how good you are,
and of your constant, daily care.
I walk in the strength of the Lord God.
I tell everyone that you alone are just and good.
O God, you have helped me from my earliest childhood -
and I have constantly testified to others
of the wonderful things you do.
And now that I am old and gray, don't forsake me.
Give me time to tell this new generation
(and their children too)
about all your mighty miracles. . . .
You have let me sink down deep in desperate problems.
But you will bring me back to life again,
up from the depths of the earth.

Psalm 71:5-20 (TLB)

NOVEMBER 27

THE WARRIOR IS A CHILD

Lately I've been winning battles left and right
But even winners can get wounded in the fight
People say that I'm amazing strong beyond my years
but they don't see inside of me - I'm hiding all the tears

They don't know that I go running home when I fall down
They don't know who picks me up when no one is around
I grab my sword and cry for just awhile
'Cause deep inside this armor the warrior is a child.

Unafraid because His armor is the best
But even soldiers need a quiet place to rest
People say that I'm amazing never face retreat
But they don't see the enemies that lay me at His feet

They don't know that I go running home when I fall down
They don't know who picks me up when no one is around
I drop my sword and look up for a smile
'Cause deep inside this armor the warrior is a child

Words and Music by Twila Paris

NOVEMBER 28

But the believers who had fled Jerusalem
went everywhere preaching the Good News about Jesus!

Philip, for instance, went to the city of Samaria
and told the people there about Christ.
Crowds listened intently to what he had to say
because of the miracles he did.

Many evil spirits were cast out,
screaming as they left their victims,
and many who were paralyzed or lame
were **healed**,

so there was much joy in that city!

Acts 8:4-8 (TLB)

NOVEMBER 29

During the 1990 Christmas season I heard anew the names of Jesus and realized that during 1990 I had experienced Jesus in each of those roles.

Isaiah 9:6 says . . . and His name will be called

WONDERFUL COUNSELOR
God told me specifically what we were to do
as I sought medical insight for Ron's illness,
leading us to Kansas City, finding a house,
finding a church that worships and prays

MIGHTY GOD
God did amazing things in our life

EVERLASTING FATHER
He gave me the everlasting Father picture to help me
visualize (see January 25 and 26)

PRINCE OF PEACE
His Peace was with us in the middle of the turmoil

~~~~~~~~~~~~~~~~~~

Behold, the virgin shall be with child, and shall bear a Son, and they shall call His Name Immanuel, which translated means, "God with us." Matthew 1:23, Isaiah 7:14 NAS

No Doubt! in 1990 God was with us!
To God be the Glory, Great Things He Has Done!
~~~~~~~~~~~~~~~~~~

NOVEMBER 30

Be strong and courageous,
do not be afraid or tremble at them,
for the Lord your God is the one who
goes with you.
He will not fail you or forsake you.

Deuteronomy 31:6 NAS

Lord, today I am feeling like this . . .

DECEMBER 1

Jesus said,

*"**Ask**, and you will be given what you ask for*

*   **Seek**, and you will find*

*   **Knock**, and the door will be opened.*

*For everyone who asks, **receives**.*

*Anyone who seeks, **finds.***

If only you will knock,

***the door will open**."*

Matthew 7:7-8 (TLB)

DECEMBER 2

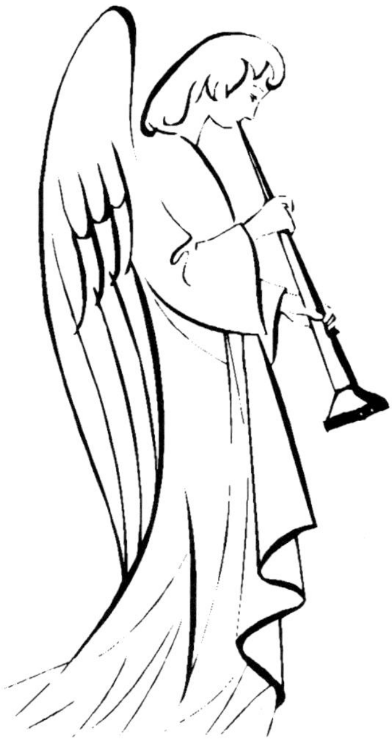

Now it came about that the poor man died and he was carried away by the angels to Abrahams bosom . . . Luke 16:22 NAS

But when we cried out to the Lord, He heard our voice
and sent an angel and brought us out from Egypt . . .
Numbers 20:16 NAS

For He will give His angels charge concerning you,
to guard you in all your ways.
They will bear you up in their hands,
lest you strike your foot against a stone.
Psalm 91:11 NAS

DECEMBER 3

Peter traveled from place to place to visit them,
and in his travels came to the believers in the town of Lydda.

There he met a man named Aeneas,
paralyzed and bedridden for eight years.

Peter said to him,
"Aeneas! Jesus Christ has healed you!
Get up and make your bed."

And he was **healed instantly**.

Then the whole population of Lydda and Sharon
turned to the Lord
when they saw Aeneas walking around.

Acts 9:32-35 (TLB)

DECEMBER 4

Rules . . . as liberating in social activity

as bones are in physical activity. . . .

Rules governing behavior work because, like bones, they are hard.

The first four of the Ten Commandments are rules governing a person's relationship to God Himself: . . .

I love you so much that I will give you Myself.
I am true reality, the only God you will ever need.
In Me alone will you find wholeness.

I desire a wonderful thing: a direct, personal relationship between Myself and each of you. You don't need inferior representation of Me, such as dead wooden idols. You can have Me. Value that.

I love you so much that I have given you My name. You will be known as "God's people" on earth. Value the privilege; don't misuse it by profaning your new name or by not living up to it.

I have given you a beautiful world to work in, play in, and enjoy. In your involvement, though, set aside a day to remember where the world came from. Your bodies need the rest; your spirits need the reminder.

The next six commandments govern personal relationships: . . .

Honor your father and mother; . . . if you do so, you shall have a long, prosperous life in the land he is giving you.

Human life is sacred. I gave it, and it has enormous worth. Cling to it. Respect it; it is the image of God. He who ignores this and commits the sacrilege of murder must be punished.

Continued on December 5

DECEMBER 5

The deepest human relationship possible is marriage. I created it to solve the essential loneliness in the heart of every person. To spread what is meant for marriage alone among a variety of people will devalue and destroy that relationship. Save sex and intimacy for its rightful place within marriage.

I am entrusting you with property. You can own things, and you should use them responsibility. Ownership is a great privilege. For it to work, you must respect everyone else's right to ownership; stealing violates that right.

I am a God of truth. Relationships only succeed when they are governed by truth. A lie destroys contracts, promises, trust. You are worthy of trust; express it by not lying.

I have given you good things to enjoy: oxen, grains, gold, furniture, musical instruments. But people are always more important than things. Love people; use things. Do not use people for your love of things.

Stripped down, the commandments emerge a basic skeleton of trust that links relationships between people and between people and God.

DECEMBER 6

CHRISTMAS HOUSE CLEANING

Part of getting ready for Christmas is a good house cleaning:

shampoo rugs . . . wash windows . . . clean cupboards . . .
wax furniture . . . get out the good dishes . . .

hard work!!

All the nooks and crannies of the house are cleaned out.
Furniture gets a fresh shine.

Now . . . I am ready for Christmas company.

But . . . **wait!!** . . . have I cleaned out all the nooks and crannies of my heart . . . the hidden sins that I don't want Jesus to see when He comes to visit??

He is the most important Christmas Company.

Am I cleaned up and ready for His visit?

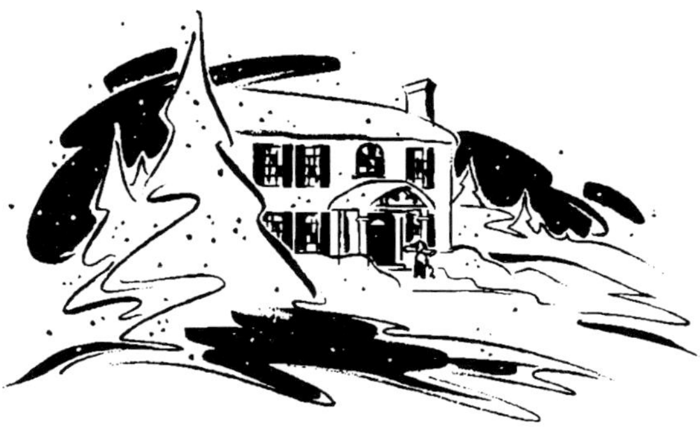

Purify me with hyssop, and I shall be clean;
Wash me, and I shall be whiter than snow.
Psalm 51:7 NAS

DECEMBER 7

When I saw their fear,
I rose and spoke to the nobles, the officials,
and the rest of the people:

"Do not be afraid of them;
remember the Lord who is great and awesome,
and fight for your brothers, your sons,
your daughters, your wives, and your houses."

Nehemiah 4:14 NAS

Lord, today I am feeling like this . . .

DECEMBER 8

Lord, you trusted Your Son to the care of earthly parents.
Fill me with Your Love to care for my loved one with the same dedication on this unknown journey.

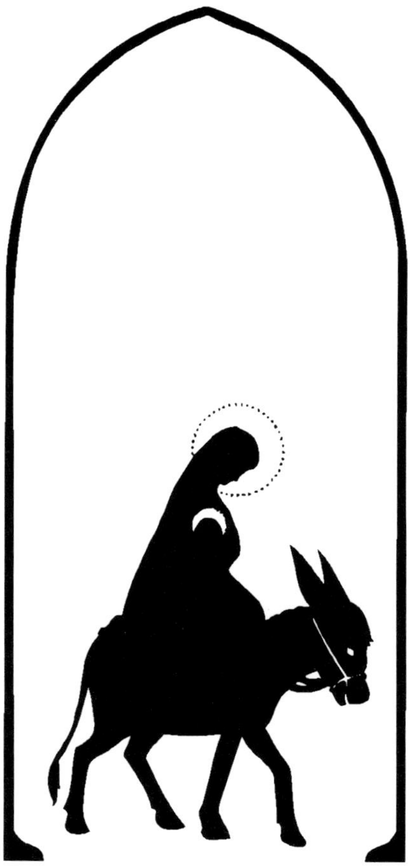

But Mary treasured up all these things,
pondering them in her heart.
Luke 2:19 NAS

DECEMBER 9

But as for me,
when they were sick,
my clothing was sackcloth;
I humbled my soul with fasting;
and my prayer kept returning to my bosom.

Psalm 35:13 NAS

Lord, today I am feeling like this . . .

DECEMBER 10

So Moses went and spoke these words to all Israel.
And he said to them,
"I am a hundred and twenty years old today;
I am no longer able to come and go,
and the LORD has said to me,
'You shall not cross this Jordan,' . . .

Be strong and courageous,
do not be afraid or tremble at them,
for the LORD your God is the one who goes WITH you.
He will not fail you or forsake you."

Then Moses called to Joshua and said to him
in the sight of all Israel,

"**Be strong and courageous**,
for you shall go with this people into the land
which the LORD has sworn to their fathers
to give them,
and you shall give it to them
as an inheritance."

Then He (Moses) commissioned Joshua . . . and said,

"**Be strong and courageous**,
for you shall bring the sons of Israel into the land
which I swore to them,
and I will be **with** you."

Deuteronomy 31:1, 2, 6-7, 23 NAS

DECEMBER 11

The LORD said to Joshua as he was ready to lead the people into the promised land:

"Be strong and courageous,
for you shall give this people possession of the land
which I swore to their fathers to give them.

Only be strong and very courageous;
be careful to do according to all the law
which Moses My servant commanded you;
do not turn from it to the right or to the left,
so that you may have success
wherever you go. . . .

Be strong and courageous!
Do not tremble or be dismayed,
for the LORD your God is with you
wherever you go." . . .

The people said to Joshua,

". . . Only be strong and courageous"

Joshua 1:6-7, 9, 18 NAS

DECEMBER 12

In the city of Joppa there was a woman named Dorcas,
a believer who was always doing kind things for others,
especially for the poor.

About this time **she became ill and died.**
Her friends prepared her for burial and
laid her in an upstairs room.

But when they learned that Peter was nearby at Lydda,
they sent two men to beg him to return with them to Joppa.
This he did; as soon as he arrived,
they took him upstairs where Dorcas lay.

The room was filled with weeping widows
who were showing one another the coats and
other garments Dorcas had made for them.
But Peter asked them all to leave the room;
then he knelt and prayed.

Turning to the body he said,
"Get up, Dorcas," and she opened her eyes!
And when she saw Peter, she sat up!

He gave her his hand and helped her up
and called in the believers and widows,
presenting her to them.

The news raced through the town,
and many believed in the Lord.

Acts 9:36-42 (TLB)

DECEMBER 13

TODAY IS SILENT DAY.

DO NOT **LOOK** at a newspaper, magazine, book,
or any printed page.

DO NOT **HEAR** television, VCR, radio, cassette tape,
or any reproduction of sound.

DO NOT **SPEAK** unnecessarily. Limit your verbal contact
with people. Unplug the telephone!

DO NOT **STAY INSIDE**. Make time today to be outside
in God's world of nature.

When o u t s i d e . . .

LOOK for God's creations in nature
HEAR what God says through nature
Let God **SPEAK** to you about the birth of His Son
for you and in you.

Christ's mortal birth
enables my immortal birth.

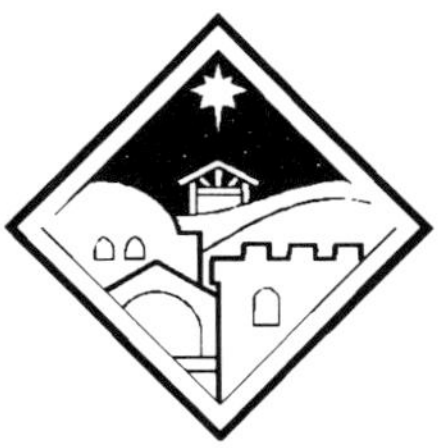

DECEMBER 14

What I want from you is your true thanks;
I want your promises fulfilled.
I want you to trust Me in your times of trouble,
so I can rescue you,
and you can give Me glory.

Psalm 50:14-15 (TLB)

Lord, today I am feeling like this . . .

DECEMBER 15

And Joseph named the first-born Manasseh,
"For," he said,
"God has made me forget all my trouble . . ."

And he named the second Ephraim,
"For," he said,
"God has made me fruitful in the land of my affliction."

Genesis 41:51-52 NAS

Lord, you are the healer of memories and the giver of new fruit in my life.
I praise you for Your healing and provisions to me.

DECEMBER 16

Our bodies have many parts,
but the many parts make up only one body
when they are all put together.
So it is with the "body" of Christ. . . .

Yes, the body has many parts, not just one part.
If the foot says, "I am not a part of the body
because I am not a hand,"
that does not make it any less a part of the body.
And what would you think if you heard an ear say,
"I am not part of the body because I am only an ear,
and not an eye?"
Would that make it any less a part of the body?
Suppose the whole body were an eye -
then how would you hear?
Or if your whole body were just one big ear,
how could you smell anything?

But that isn't the way God has made us.
He has made many parts for our bodies
and has put each part just where he wants it.

What a strange thing a body would be if it had only one part!
So he has made many parts, but still there is only one body.
The eye can never say to the hand, "I don't need you."
The head can't say to the feet, "I don't need you."

And some of the parts that seem weakest and
least important are really the most necessary.
Yes, we are especially glad to have some parts
that seem rather odd!
And we carefully protect from the eyes of others
those parts that should not be seen,
while of course the parts that may be seen
do not require this special care.

Continued on December 17

DECEMBER 17

So God has put the body together in such a way that extra honor and care are given to those parts that might otherwise seem less important.

This makes for happiness among the parts,
so that the parts have the same care for each other
that they do for themselves.

If one part suffers, all parts suffer with it.
And if one part is honored, all the parts are glad.

Now here is what I am trying to say:

All of you together are the one body of Christ
and each one of you is a separate and necessary part of it.

Here is a list of some of the parts He has placed in His Church, which is His body:

Apostles,
Prophets - those who preach God's Word,
Teachers,
Those who do miracles,
Those who have the gift of healing,
Those who can help others,
Those who can get others to work together,
Those who speak in languages they have never learned.

1 Corinthians 12:12-29 (TLB)

Lord, as I care for the body of my loved one, fill me with your gift of love. Open me to receive the loving and helping gifts from other members of the Body of Christ.

DECEMBER 18

No, dear brothers, I am still not all I should be
but I am bringing all my energies to bear
on this one thing:

Forgetting the past and
looking forward to what lies ahead,
I strain to reach the end of the race and
receive the prize for which God is calling us
up to heaven because of what
Christ Jesus did for us.

Philippians 3:13-14 (TLB)

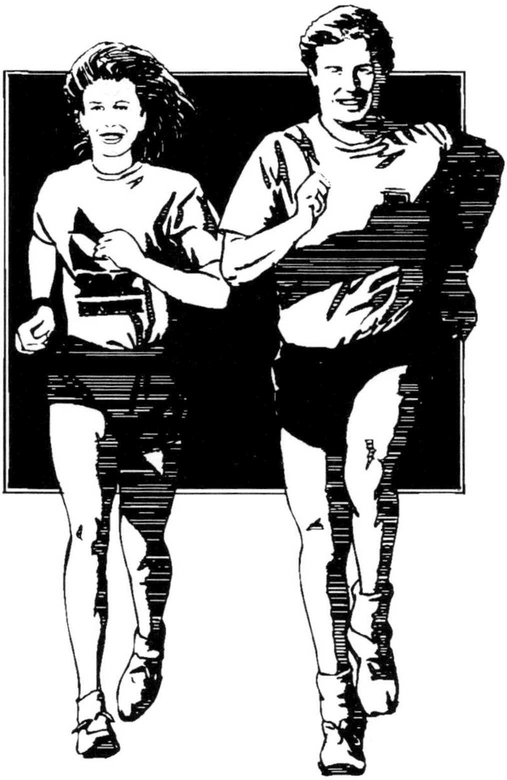

DECEMBER 19

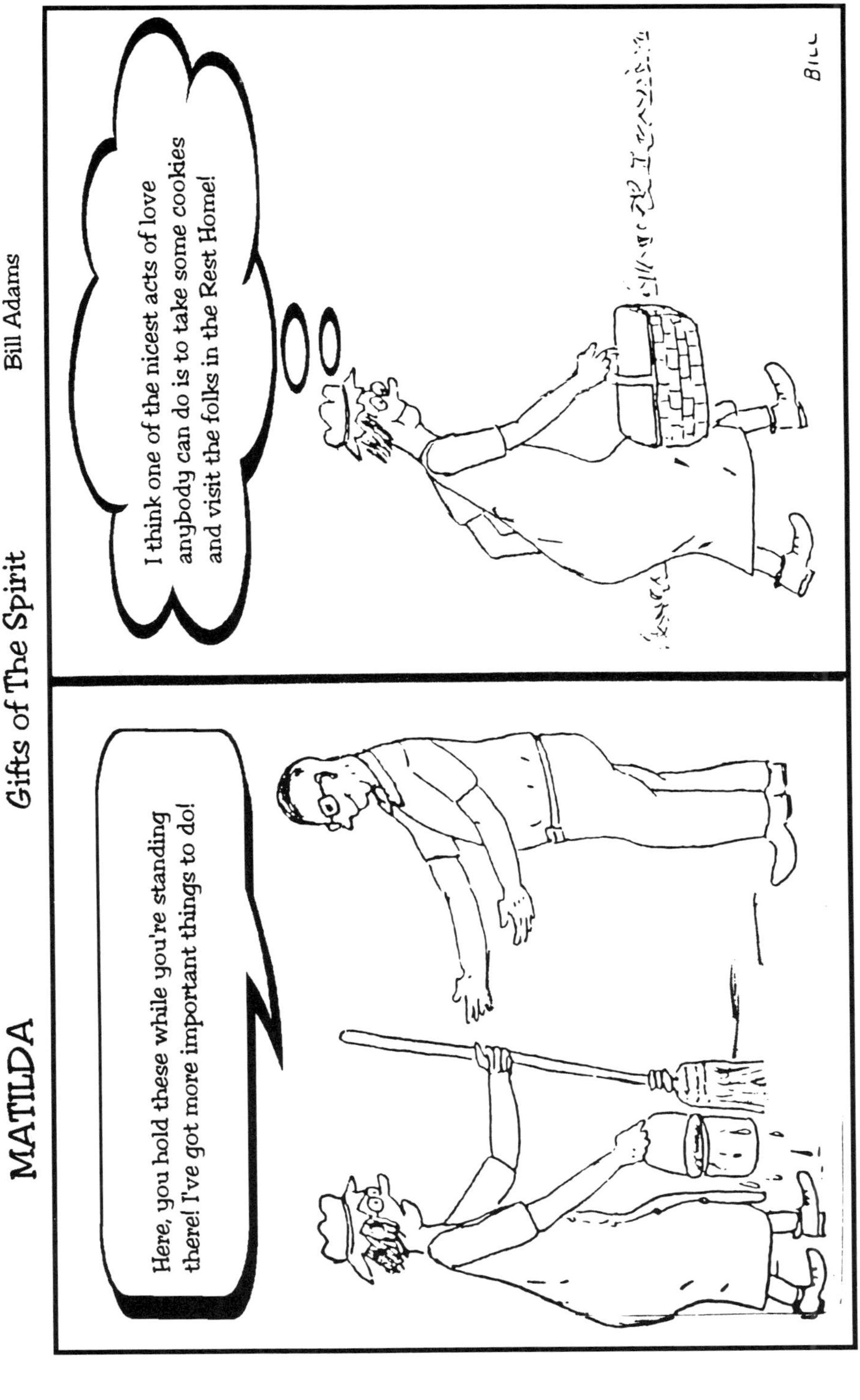
MATILDA
Gifts of The Spirit
Bill Adams
Here, you hold these while you're standing there! I've got more important things to do!
I think one of the nicest acts of love anybody can do is to take some cookies and visit the folks in the Rest Home!
BILL

DECEMBER 20

. . . Only in returning to me

and waiting for me will you be saved;

in quietness and confidence is your strength . . .

Isaiah 30:15 (TLB)

Lord, today I am feeling like this . . .

DECEMBER 21

FEAR KEEPS OUT JOY

My husband's greatest joy was to make many wooden cars and animals in his wood shop. Then, just before Christmas, he dressed as Santa Claus and made surprise deliveries to families with young children.

The summer of 1990 we moved from a small rural community where we were well known, and Santa's visits were eagerly awaited. Now we live in a large city, and I immediately saw the difference when Santa made his unannounced visits. Some people would not open the door and let Santa in. I could understand their fear of opening their door to a stranger.

I then began to see the little fears in my life that keep my door shut, locking out **Christ's joy and love.**

Lord, I say **"No!"** to **fear** and **I O P E N the door of my** heart to say **"Yes!"** to **You**. I O P E N the door and let You come into my life.

Set me free of the fears that lock out God's JOY.

This was written on December 21, 1990,
one year to the day before Ron's death.

DECEMBER 22

Although He (Jesus) was a Son (of God),

He learned obedience from the things

which He suffered.

Hebrews 5:8 NAS

Lord, today I am feeling like this . . .

What am I learning through this suffering?

DECEMBER 23

Lord, send an angel who understands me.

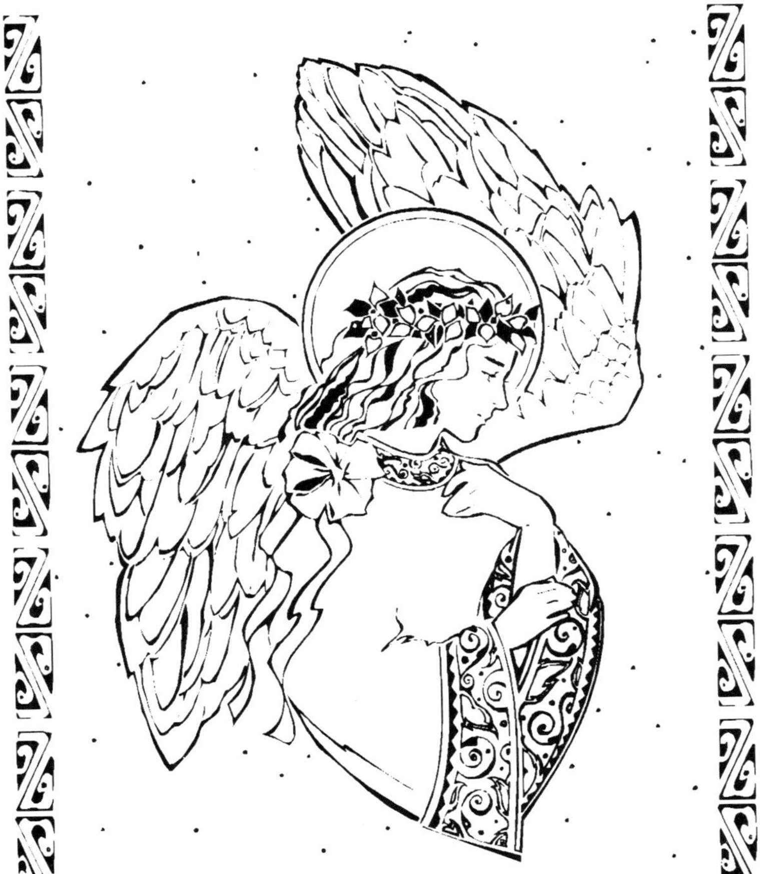

Day of Ron's Burial and Memorial Worship Service

DECEMBER 24

Christmas Eve day, 1979, was not going well. Betsy was an angry sixth grader. She was having a bad day. No amount of listening, teasing, love, correction, or threats could bring her out of her bad mood. It got so bad, we were ready to postpone our family's Christmas gift exchange scheduled to begin after attending the Christmas Eve service.

But, we were going to the annual 11:00 P.M. Christmas Eve service at Church. That was one family tradition that would not be changed, even if she didn't want to go.

Betsy sang in the Wesley Choir. They wore their robes and shared during the candlelight service. The special service, the beauty of the sanctuary, the joy of singing with a full congregation about Jesus' birth, the miracle of candlelight opened her heart and allowed the Holy Spirit to touch her with healing.

Standing in the hallway after the service with all the other Wesley Choir members, holding their candles, her eyes were aglow and she looked at me and said, "This is so pretty - I'm glad I came. I'm sorry I acted so bad at home." Praise the Lord! for God's love that heals a hurt heart. Christ was born anew in her through that Christmas Eve Service.

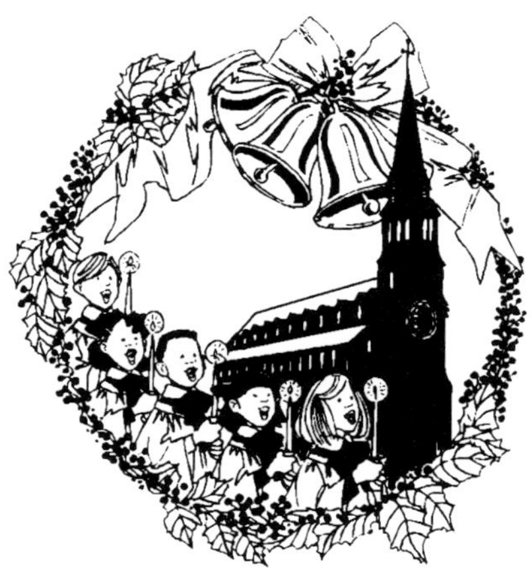

DECEMBER 25

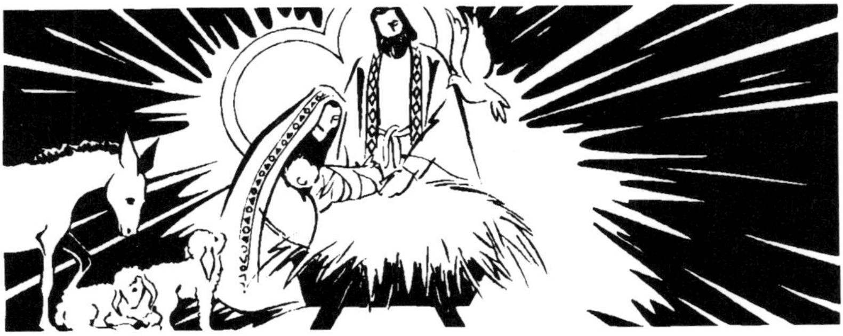

The people who walk in darkness
Will see a great light;
Those who live in a dark land,
The light will shine on them. . . .

For a child will be born to us,
a son will be given to us;
And the government will rest on His shoulders;

And His name will be called

WONDERFUL
COUNSELOR
MIGHTY GOD
ETERNAL FATHER
PRINCE OF PEACE

Isaiah 9:2, 6 NAS

DECEMBER 26

During Christmas, 1990, someone had carelessly discarded their fireplace ashes, causing a fire in a house that we pass on our way to church. There was extensive damage, and the house sat hopeless-looking all winter.

Spring brought activity around the house.

The house was demolished, leaving only the foundation and the fireplace chimney. What a mess the yard was during this phase of work!

Eventually, piles of new lumber and supplies appeared on the lawn. And soon reconstruction began.

Rebuilding can take place upon a firm foundation.

There is a season of original tragedy,
then waiting while behind the scene,
plans, estimates, ordering, etc., take place.
Time to clean up the mess.
Then delivery of new materials,
and reconstruction begins!
And eventually a house becomes a home.

Lord, right now I feel like a burned house.
Come, Holy Spirit, Come - rebuild me on my firm foundation.
I accept the pounding and rewiring of the reconstruction.
And I'll open the new door and let You live inside, also.

Can they revive the stones from the
dusty rubble - even the burned ones?
Nehemiah 4:2 NAS

DECEMBER 27

The righteous **cry**

and the Lord **hears,**

and delivers them out

of all their troubles.

The Lord is near to the brokenhearted,

And saves those who are crushed in spirit.

Many are the afflictions of the righteous;

But the Lord delivers him out of them all.

Psalm 34:17-19 NAS

DECEMBER 28

Before you put away the cards that came to your home this Christmas season, line them up on the table to tell the Christmas story.

Look at the Mary and Joseph pictures. What are Mary and Joseph saying to each other? What are they doing?

What emotion do you see on the faces of the shepherds? Fear, wonder, excitement, urgency? What are they saying at the manger?

What animals do you see in the manger scene? Lions, tigers, and bears? Or do you see the animals that are small, silent, serving, and peaceful?

What posture do all the people and animals take?

And the angels. What are they doing?

As you look at the cards and think about these questions, which person or part of the story do you most identify with right now? Who are you in the story?

All of these people and postures direct us to the way we should come to the Christmas season.

Come . . . silently . . . kneeling . . . peaceful . . . adoring . . . slowly . . . quietly . . . single mindedly . . . listening . . . looking for the still small voice of God to speak to each of us and be born anew in our heart this Christmas.

O Come, All Ye Faithful

DECEMBER 29

HOME FREE

I'm trying hard not to think You unkind
But heavenly Father, You know my heart
Surely You could read my mind
Good people underneath a sea of grief
Some get up and walk away
Some will find ultimate relief

Out in the corridor We're praying for life
A mother for her baby A husband for his wife
O, Sometimes the good die young
It's sad but true
And while we pray for one more heart beat
The real comfort is with You

We know pain has little mercy
That suffering is no respecter of age
Or race or position
I know every prayer gets answered
But the hardest one to pray is slow to come
O, Lord, not mine
But Your will be done
O, let it be

Home Free ---Eventually
At the ultimate healing
We will be Home Free
Home Free
I've gotta feeling At the ultimate healing
We will be
HOME
FREE

Words and Music by Wayne Watson

We had this sung at the Memorial Worship Service for Ron.

DECEMBER 30

THANK YOU

I dreamed I went to Heaven, and you were there with me.
We walked upon the streets of gold, beside the crystal sea.
We heard the angels singing, then someone called your name.
You turned and saw this young man, and he was smiling as he came.

And he said,

"Friend you may not know me now," and then he said
"but wait, you used to teach my Sunday School,
when I was only eight. And every week you would say a
prayer, before the class would start.
And one day when you said that prayer,
I asked Jesus in my heart."

"Thank you for giving to the Lord, I am a life that was changed,
Thank you for giving to the Lord, I am so glad you gave."

Then another one stood before you and said,

"Remember the time a missionary came to your church,
and his pictures made you cry. You didn't have much
money, but you gave it anyway. Jesus took the gift you
gave, and that's why I'm here today."

One by one they came, as far as the eye could see. Each life somehow touched, by your generosity. Little things that you had done, sacrifices made unnoticed on the earth, In Heaven now proclaimed.

And I know up in Heaven, you're not suppose to cry. But I am almost sure, there were tears in your eyes. As Jesus took your hand and you stood before the Lord, He said,

"My child, look around you, Great is your reward."

DECEMBER 31

Finally, brethren,

rejoice,

be made complete,

be comforted,

be like-minded,

live in peace;

and the God of love and peace

shall be with you.

Greet one another with a holy kiss.

All the saints greet you.

The grace of the Lord Jesus Christ,

and the love of God,

and the fellowship of the Holy Spirit,

be with you all.

2 Corinthians 13:11-14 NAS

POST SCRIPT

On Tuesday, December 10, eleven days before Ron died, he dressed for church and went to the car ready to "go." I drove to our church. We went in. The sanctuary was dark. But there was a spotlight on **two angels**, huge six-foot white angels, over the platform. It was a breathtaking moment! A complete surprise because the angels were not there on Sunday. Ron went to our spot, sat down, looked, put his head down. I sat in the back of the sanctuary to watch what would happen. After forty-five minutes I went up to him and offered him my hand to leave. It was like he did not see me. I waited another half hour. Then he was ready to go.

On Thursday, December 12, we went with our son Steve and his family to the Raytown First Baptist Church Christmas Pageant. When the angel visitation in the shepherd's scene came, it was another breathtaking moment. All of a sudden, what before had been a Bethlehem painted backdrop behind the stage, lit up with intense brilliance, and there was a handsome male angel surrounded by many female angels singing "Glory, Glory, Glory." **Immediately** Ron was up and out of there. No talking him out of it, no conversation, no way to know what was going through his mind.

We took Ron to the hospital late Thursday, December 19. On Friday, one of Steve's friends sent a homemade quilt angel to the hospital. We hung it on the IV rack over his bed.

God used angels to minister to us at our deepest time of grief. I can't wait to hear from Ron what he experienced with angels!!

FACE TO FACE

In September, 1992, I was blessed to go to Prayer and Prophetic Conferences with a group from my church. These Conferences were held in Nuremberg and Berlin, Germany.

On the last night of the Conference in Nuremberg one of the pastors had a word for me. He said,

"You are alone, but not alone. Read Isaiah 57:1-2. I can tell you that your husband is home with God, **face to face**. You are feeling warm oil of Holy Spirit. You will not have any more emptiness and lonliness from this night forward."

> The righteous man perishes, and no man takes it to heart;
> And devout men are taken away, while no one understands.
> For the righteous man is taken away from evil,
> He enters into peace; they rest in their beds,
> Each one who walked in his upright way. Isaiah 57:1-2 NAS

In October, 1992, I was back in Greenfield, Ohio, visiting family and friends. One afternoon I was sitting with a friend sharing some of my remaining grief emotions, especially about Ron's last days because he was so confused.

As I cried and we talked and and prayed this through, the Holy Spirit gave my friend 1 Corinthians 13, the Love Chapter. She read it aloud. When she read the twelfth verse - instantly - major peace flooded my emotions. I was **set free** by this truth.

> For now we see in a mirror dimly, but then **face to face**;
> now I know in part, but then I shall know fully
> just as I also have been fully known.

Yes, Ron was confused here on earth. But because he is now **face to face** with the Lord, he now **knows** and now he has peace.

TWO ANGELS

In the movie, *It's a Wonderful Life,* the opening scene is the prayers of all the people in a town going up for George because something is wrong with him. They are prayers from people whose lives were changed because he lived a life of servant love. We are shown scenes from all seasons of his life. We see his hopes and dreams as a youth. We watch as he denies himself - time after time - to give his whole life to others. We watch as these people continually live their own self-centered lives - better because George had a part in it. We watch him continually "fix" others' mistakes and stand up with courage against the evil in the town. Even to the point of taking personal responsibility for others' mistakes.

UNTIL

the load on his shoulders and in his heart is more than he can bear. He does turn to You, God. The intercessory prayers of George's family and friends for him reach You. And You send an angel named Clarence (was my dad's name) to rescue George and bring him back to reality.

When he does go home, he finds all his friends and family pouring out their love on him as their eyes and hearts have been opened to see and appreciate his role in their lives.

Lord, Ron experienced that same outpouring of love at his retirement dinner in Greenfield. We heard testimony after testimony of Ron's influence in people's lives.

Could he **hear**, Lord? Did he **know**, Lord?!

He dreamed of being a golf pro. But he, too, married, raised a family, "fathered" athletes, and was "Santa" to many children.

And he cried out "WHY? WHY? WHY?"

The prayers of Ron's family and worldwide friends went up in intercession to You, Lord. And

You Heard.

You sent **TWO ANGELS** to bring him home to work with You.

To live in Your Crystal City with all Your little children.

And the many saints in Kansas City, Greenfield, and Greenmont in Dayton, Ohio gathered to praise You for his earthly life.

Lord, Ron's presence is everywhere in this Christmas house.

In the wood ornaments on our tree that he made
In the wood JESUS he made that sits on my mantle
In the Santa in his sleigh and the Santa kneeling
before Jesus that sit on my mantle
In the train village beneath the tree
In the sound of shop tools as our sons work in the
basement wood shop
In the ornaments that Ron put on our first tree that
he surprised me with 34 years ago

and in the row of angels that hang in the window above my nativity - one for each family member.

But, Ron's wooden angel hangs on the front door wreath that has bells on it. And every time the door is opened - the bells ring.

And I'm reminded that another angel has gotten his wings at Christmas - just as Ron did last year at this time.

Thank you, Lord, for **two angels**!!

Written Friday, December 18, 1992, one year after Ron's death.

GRIEVING

Through this past year of grieving, I **have learned** that grief comes in waves . . . some tiny - that just swirl around my ankles - some major - that almost drown me, and I come up sputtering and thrashing. I **have learned**, also, that the Lord has a **truth** and **healing** in each wave.

After a year, I can see now how much healing God has done in my life. Last year, peace that passes understanding (Philippians 4:7) became alive in my heart. This year it is the Joy of the Lord (Jeremiah 31:13). As I came up to the anniversary of Ron's Homegoing, I came with the joy of the Lord that has replaced my mourning.

On December 18th a **major grief wave** came upon me. I rode it through and processed the truths God wanted me to learn. After the wave, the Two Angels prayer came forth.

Now a couple weeks later, I also see how God has used others to go before and prepare the way. I want to share this with you to encourage you as you live out you own loving life with others.

Sue Ann, about four years ago at Christmas, gave each of the gals in the office a gold bell on a chain.

Ethel Ann commented when she saw me wearing the bell that an angel had just gotten its wings. I didn't know what she meant. She told me about the movie *It's a Wonderful Life*. Then she took the extra step to record it when it was on TV and give the tape to me. I didn't get to watch it until Christmas of 1990. I watched it again with Steve's family at Christmas of '91 and '92.

Mindy, Christmas 1988, gave Ron a Santa kneeling before the Baby Jesus in the manager knowing that it was God's love in Ron's heart that motivated him to make toys and surprise Santa visits to her children.

Tim gave Ron a Santa in a sleigh at Ron's retirement dinner in June, 1990 because he was so touched by the years of Santa visits to his children.

A young father here in Kansas City was in prayer for Ron the night we took him to the hospital. The Lord gave him this vision . . . "**Two angels**, with wings and everything, bright and powerful looking. Between them, I saw Ron, with a **huge smile** on his face, looking upward between and past the angels. **He was not looking at the angels, rather, he was definitely looking upward past the angels. His arms were raised, stretched up towards where he was looking.** I can still see this picture in my mind. Ron was overjoyed, happy and he definitely knew where he was going, and it appeared that he was quite happy about it. I got the distinct impression that he was rising upwards with the angels."

In several earlier dreams the Lord had given me, there were glass rooms/houses and all had little children in them. I knew I was seeing small glimpses of Ron's heavenly home.

Intercessory prayer, dreams, visions, and angels are all new dimensions of God's personal working in our life that the Lord has taught me through this sorrow and suffering. I wanted to share these brief glimpses of how God used the faithful prayers and gifts given to us.

Peace I leave with you; My peace I give to you;
not as the world gives, do I give to you.
Let not your heart be troubled, nor let it be fearful.
You heard that I said to you,
'I go away and I will come to you.'
If you loved Me, you would have rejoiced,
because I go to the Father; for the Father is greater than I.
And now I have told you before it came to pass,
that when it comes to pass you may believe.
John 14:27-29 NAS

This was the *Upper Room Devotional* reading on the day I was proofreading and editing this page. Now I realize why God gave me all the supernatural experiences before Ron died. I do now believe because I have seen and experienced God's love and grace and comfort.

This letter was written January 2, 1993 to the friends mentioned.

12 Step Program Can Help Caregivers

The Twelve Step Program was originally developed as the heart of the Alcoholics Anonymous program in order to provide a unity of purpose and guidance for individual growth. Today many self-help groups have adapted these twelve steps for various purposes.

STEP 1: I can control how the disease affects me and my family.
Caregivers should acknowledge those aspects over which they have no control. Ultimately, no matter what the caregiver does, the disease process will not change. Some caregivers have reported that the Serenity Prayer has been helpful to them. It is as follows:
"God, grant me the serenity to accept the things I cannot change,
the courage to change the things I can change,
and the wisdom to know the difference."

STEP 2: I need to take care of myself.
Caregivers need to give themselves permission to "indulge" in such things as obtaining relief by using respite resources and by involvement in outside activities that they both need and enjoy.

STEP 3: I need to simplify my lifestyle.
If a caregiver wishes to maintain outside activities and interests, he or she will need to lower unrealistic expectations they may have of themselves.

STEP 4: I need to allow others to help me.
Caregivers often report that friends say, "Call me if you need help." The caregiver should keep a list of activities nearby, and when this offer is made he or she can say, "I need help with . . . "

STEP 5: I need to take one day at a time.
This slogan is borrowed directly from Alcoholics Anonymous and is used often by family caregivers. For the person with dementia, it is essentially the "here and now" that is significant - a reality to which caregivers must adapt.

STEP 6: I need to structure my day.
Routine and structure may give the family member a greater sense of safety and security, and the caregiver will be able to use his or her time more efficiently.

STEP 7: I need to have a sense of humor.
Maintaining a sense of humor means that caregivers have to be objective enough to see the irony in painful situations. One caregiver said, "I choose to make this a humorous heartache."

STEP 8: I need to remember that my relative's behavior and emotions are distorted by his or her illness.

STEP 9: I need to focus on and enjoy what my relative can still do.
Enjoying the good moments for what they provide is commonly seen by caregivers as a way of helping themselves through their present difficulties.

STEP 10: I need to depend on other relationships for love and support.
A desire to be cared about and supported by others is a normal human response, and it is essential to have these needs met in some way.

STEP 11: I need to remind myself that I am doing the best I can at this very moment.
It is important for the caregivers to acknowledge their human limitations, develop a sense of acceptance of themselves, and accept how they have managed a particular situation.

STEP 12: A Higher Power is available to me. (God)
This step does not suggest imposing a set of beliefs on other people, but does encourage caregivers to develop their own concept of a Higher Power that may work in their own lives as caregivers.

Courtesy of the Wyoming Chapter Newsletter
Greater Kansas City Area Chapter Alzheimer's Association
Awareness Newsletter, January/February, 1996

WORKS CITED

ART WORK

My drawings using Ami Pro 2.0, Samna Corp, Lotus Development Corporation, Aug 15, Sept 22, 24.

Mary Bruno illustrations, Jan 1, 2, 18; Feb 21; Mar 28, 31; Apr 24, 30; May 31; June 9; July 18; Sept 20, 29; Oct 6; Nov 17, 24.

Pat Jessee illustrations for *With Open Hands*, 1972 edition, are adapted from original photographs by Theo Robert.

All other graphics reproduced using: ClickArt ® Image Pak™ ; © Broderbund Software, Inc. All Rights Reserved. Used By Permission.

AUTHOR UNKNOWN

Jan 13	Healing of Memories Prayer
Jan 18	Hugging
May 31	Pedal
Sept 4	Prayer of St. Francis of Assisi, A Modern Translation

BIBLES

NAS	Scripture quotations marked NAS are taken from the NEW AMERICAN STANDARD BIBLE ®, © Copyright The Lockman Foundation 1960, 1962, 1963, 1968, 1971, 1972, 1973, 1975, 1977. Used by permission.
NIV	Scripture quotations marked NIV are adapted from the *Holy Bible, New International Version. NIV.* Copyright 1973, 1978, 1984 by International Bible Society. All rights reserved.
TLB	Scripture quotations marked (TLB) are taken from *The Living Bible* copyright © 1971. Used by permission of Tyndale House Publishers, Inc., Wheaton, Illinois 60189. All rights reserved.

BOOKS

Jan 7, Feb 6, Jul 30

From: *Doorposts.* By: Timothy Botts © 1986. Used by permission of Tyndale House Publishers, Inc. All rights reserved. Scripture References from *The Living Bible* © 1971.

Apr 25, May 17, 18, Aug 20, 21

From: *Windsongs.* By: Timothy Botts © 1989. Used by permission of Tyndale House Publishers, Inc. All rights reserved.

Dec 4, 5 — Brand, Paul and Philip Yancey. *Fearfully & Wonderfully Made.* Copyright © 1980. Used by permission of Zondervan Publishing House.

Nov 7 — Brand, Paul and Philip Yancey. *In His Image.* Copyright © 1984. Used by permission of Zondervan Pushlishing House.

Feb 26,27,28 — Excerpted from TEAMMATES by Bruce Cook and Howard Henricks. Copyright 1987, Leadership Dynamics Interntional. All rights reserved. Used by permission of Walk Thru the Bible, 4201 N. Peachtree Road, Atlanta, GA 30341. 1-770-458-9300, Ext. 212

May 3-5 — From: *Hinds' Feet On High Places,* By: Hannah Hurnard © 1975 by Tyndale House Publishers, Inc. Used by permission. All rights reserved.

Apr 3, Jun 18 — Nouwen, Henri J. M. *The Road to Daybreak,* Copyright © 1988 by Henri J. M. Nouwen. Used by permission of Doubleday, a division of Bantam Doubleday Dell Publishing Group, Inc.

Oct 1, 8, 14, 22, 30, Nov 5, 12

Nouwen, Henri J. M., *With Open Hands*, © 1972, 1995. Ave Maria Press. Used with permission. All Rights Reserved. Illustrations adapted from original photographs by Theo Robert.

CARTOONS, DRAWINGS, PHOTOGRAPHS

Apr 10	Adams, Bill, *Matilda*
Dec 19	Adams, Bill, *Matilda*
Cover	Crusie, Dan, *Set Free*
July 22	Johnston, Lynn, *For Better or For Worse*, 9-23-90, © Lynn Johnston Productions Inc./Dist. by United Feature Syndicate, Inc.
Mar 12	Keane, Bil, *The Family Circus Treasury*, copyright 1977 by Bil Keane. Reprinted with special permission of the King Features Syndicate.
Mar 14	Sims, Sharon, *Light in Darkness*
Jan 25	Wood, Shannon, *Everlasting Arms*
July 25	Wood, Steve, *Woodland Acres Shelter House*
Feb 14	Wedding Picture, Photographer Unknown
Feb 17	Hands on Bible, Photographer Unknown
June 4	Greenfield Aerial, Photographer Unknown

MUSIC

Mar 27	Ackley, Alfred H., *He Lives,* The Rodeheaver Co., © 1933 Renewed 1961 The Rodeheaver Co. (A Div. of WORD MUSIC) All Rights Reserved. Used by Permission.
Dec 30	Boltz, Ray, Words and Music. *Thank You.* Copyright ©1988, Gaither Music. All Rights Reserved.
Sept 26	Crouch, Andrae. *Through It All.* Copyright 1971by Manna Music, Inc., 35255 Brooten Road, Pacific City, OR 97135. All Rights Reserved. Used by Permission. (ASCAP)
Jun 12	Kaiser, Kurt. *Pass It On*, Bud-John Songs Inc., © 1969. All Rights reserved. Used by Permision. P O Box 5085, Brentwood TN 37024.
Nov 27	Paris, Twila. *Warrior is a Child,* © 1984 Singspiration Music/ASCAP. All Rights Reserved. Used by Permission of Brentwood-Benson Music Publishing, Inc.
July 11	Rodgers, Richard and Hammerstein II, Oscar. *You'll Never Walk Alone*, © 1945 (Renewed) Williamson Music, International Copyright Secured, Reprinted by Permission, All Rights Reserved.

July 8	Scott, Clara, "Open My Eyes That I May See." Page 454 from *The United Methodist Hymnal.* © 1989, The Methodist Publishing House.
Sept 17	Spafford, Horatio G., Philip P. Bliss, "It is Well With My Soul." Page 377 from *The United Methodist Hymnal.* © 1989, The Methodist Publishing House.
Sept 10	Warner, Anna B., William B. Bradbury, "Jesus Loves Me." Page 191 from *The United Methodist Hymnal.* © 1989, The Methodist Publishing House.
Dec. 29	Watson, Wayne. *Home Free,* © 1990 Word Music (A Div. of WORD MUSIC), Material Music (Admin. By WORD MUSIC). All Rights Reserved. Used By Permision.

WRITINGS FROM OTHERS

Mar 6	Campbell, Bob, *Pastor's Ice Prayer*
Sept 12	Grant, Alan, *The Difference*
Aug 2	Niebuhr, Reinhold, *Serenity Prayer*

BOOKS THAT BLESSED ME IN THIS SEASON BUT NOT CITED IN THIS CAREGIVERS JOURNAL

Dunnam, Maxie. *The Workbook of Intercessory Prayer.* Nashville, The Upper Room, 1979.

The Workbook of Living Prayer. Nashville, The Upper Room, 1974.

Teague, Sam E., *The John Wesley - Great Experiment.* Nashville, Spiritual Life Publishers Inc. 1965.

Flynn, *Mister God, this is Anna.* New York: Holt, Rinehart and Winston.

Graham, Billy, *Angels, God's Secret Agents.* Doubleday and Company, Inc., Garden City, New York, 1975

Malz, Betty. *Angels Watching Over Me.* Old Tappan: Chosen Books, Fleming H. Revell Co., 1986

INDEX

JESUS HEALINGS

OLD TESTAMENT

Feb 8/9	Genesis 1-2	Creation
Aug 5	Genesis 15:1	Do Not Fear
Dec 15	Genesis 41:51-52	Joseph, Son's Names
Feb 11	Exodus 3:12	Mountaintop
July 14	Exodus 14:13-22	Red Sea
May 1	Exodus 15:24-27	Lord Is Healer
Mar 24	Exodus 17:10-12	Moses Arms Tired
June 26	Exodus 23:20-30	Little by Little
July 7	Exodus 35-36	Craftsman
Mar 2	Numbers 6:22-27	Blessings
Nov 21	Numbers 9:8	Wait, Listen
Dec 2	Numbers 20:16	Angel
Aug 5	Numbers 21:34	Do Not Fear
July 11, Nov 30	Deuteronomy 31:6	Be Strong and Courageous
Dec 10	Deuteronomy 31 verses	Be Strong and Courageous
Jan 26	Deuteronomy 33:27	Everlasting Arms
Dec 11	Joshua 1:6-7, 9, 18	Be Strong And Courageous
June 6	Joshua 6:1-22	March Around
May 8	Joshua 24:15	But as for Me
July 5	Joshua 24:15	Choose Today
Nov 4	1 Samuel 17	David/Goliath
Mar 8/9	2 Samuel 12:16-24	Child Died
Aug 6	2 Samuel 17:28,29	People
Aug 26	2 Samuel 17:28,29	Brought Supplies
Oct 15/16	2 Kings 5:1-15	Naaman
Jan 14	2 Kings 6:16	Do Not Fear
Aug 12	2 Kings 20:1-11	Three People/Three Things
Nov 13	1 Chronicles 12:22	Army of God
Jan 11	2 Chronicles 7:12-16	Humble, Pray
Jan 3	2 Chronicles 7:14	Early Morning
Jan 28	2 Chronicles 15:7	Be Strong
Apr 13	2 Chronicles 6:9	Down/Up
June 13/14	2 Chronicles 20:1-30	Battle Is Lord's
Nov 15	2 Chronicles 32:7	One With Us Is Greater
Dec 7	Nehemiah 4:14	Do Not Be Afraid
June 30	Esther 2:7	Adopted
Nov 16	Job 2:11-13	Friends Came
Mar 7	Job 14:7-9	Hope for Tree
Feb 16	Job 23, 27 verses	Gold
Mar 18	Job 23:10-12	Come Forth as Gold
Sept 6	Job 33:12-30	Dreams, Sickness, Angel
Jan 17	Job 42:1-6	Why?

May 8	Psalm 5:7	But As for Me
Mar 11	Psalm 6:2-10	Heal Me
Apr 9	Psalm 16:7	Counsel
Mar 20	Psalm 20	Prayer for Caregivers
Aug 29	Psalm 23	Lord Is Shepherd
Apr 2	Psalm 23:4	Bitter or Better
Mar 25	Psalm 25:4-7, 16-21	My Hope Is in You
May 8	Psalm 26:11,12	But as for Me
Mar 15	Psalm 27:1,4-7	Light in Darkness
June 30, Oct 31	Psalm 27:10	Lord Take Me Up
Sept 30	Psalm 27:4-7, 13-14	House of Lord
Oct 13	Psalm 28:6-9	Bless Lord
Aug 19	Psalm 30	Joy in Morning
Apr 8	Psalm 30:2-5	Joy in Morning
June 29	Psalm 31:14-15	Times in God's Hand
July 21	Psalm 31:9-16, 20	Depression
July 24	Psalm 31:20,21	Shelter
Apr 1	Psalm 32:3-5,7-8.11	Silent Sin
Sept 5	Psalm 32:7-9	Stubborn Mule
Oct 21	Psalm 33	Sing For Joy
Oct 18	Psalm 34:7	Angel
Dec 27	Psalm 34:17-19	Lord Hears
May 8, Dec 9	Psalm 35:13	But as for Me
Apr 15	Psalm 40:1-3, 8,17	Wait Patiently
Sept 23	Psalm 41:1-3	Lord Sustain
Feb 18	Psalm 45:13	King's Daughter
Oct 29	Psalm 46	God Is Refuge
Dec 14	Psalm 50:14-15	Give God Glory
May 8	Psalm 52:8,9	But as for Me
Aug 24	Psalm 55:16-18	Evening, Morning, Noon
July 29	Psalm 66:16-20	I Cried, He Listened
Nov 26	Psalm 71:5-20	Trusted from Childhood
Sept 16	Psalm 81	Relieved Shoulder
Aug 6	Psalm 91:11,12	Protection
Dec 2	Psalm 91:11	Angel
Oct 7	Psalm 107	Sacrifices of Thanksgiving
Nov 20	Psalm 116:1-15	Precious Is Saints' Death
Jan 4	Psalm 119	Word
Apr 9	Psalm 119:12-20	Word
Oct. 4	Psalm 119:24	Laws Counselors
Mar 17	Psalm 119:28	Weep With Grief
Mar 10	Psalm 119:92	Law Delight
Sept 18	Psalm 119:105	Word Lamp
Sept 13	Psalm 130:5	Soul Waits
Nov 19	Psalm 139:13-18, 23-24	You Made Me

Oct 17	Proverbs 1:5	Wise Man
Nov 11	Proverbs 3:1-12	Wisdom/Why
June 20	Proverbs 4:20-27	Whole Body Health
May 9	Proverbs 6:16-19	Lord Hates
Jan 16	Proverbs 16:11	Just Balance
July 13	Ecclesiastes 3:7	Listen/Silent
Aug 6	Song of Solomon 4:7,9	Passion
Feb 4	Song of Solomon 4:11-12	Valley
May 25	Isaiah 6:1-3	Worship at Death
Nov 29	Isaiah 9:6	His Name
Dec 25	Isaiah 9:2,6	See Light
Oct 6	Isaiah 11:2	Spirit of Lord
July 6, Dec 20	Isaiah 30:15	Quietness Is Strength
May 12	Isaiah 33:2,14-16	Strength Every Morning
Apr 23	Isaiah 35:1-7	Wilderness/Desert
Jan 24	Isaiah 40:31	Eagles Wings
Mar 4	Isaiah 40:31	Wait
Jan 31	Isaiah 43:1-5	Through Waters
Aug 10	Isaiah 43:4	Precious
Sept 2	Isaiah 43:18-21	Rivers in Desert
June 30	Isaiah 49:15-16	Inscribed on Palms
Mar 26	Isaiah 53:5	His Wounds
Oct 31	Isaiah 53:6	Astray
Aug 24	Isaiah 56:7	House of Prayer
Nov 10	Isaiah 57:1,2	Righteous Man
June 22	Isaiah 58:11	Bones
Sept 9	Isaiah 61:1-4,7,10	Spirit of Lord on Me
Feb 21	Isaiah 63:9	Angel
Sept 27	Isaiah 65:24	Before Call
Aug 5	Jeremiah 1:8	Do Not Be Afraid
Jan 21	Jeremiah 30:17	Restore Health, Heal
Aug 31	Jeremiah 31:13	Mourning Into Joy
May 19	Lamentations 3:19-26	Great Is Thy Faithfulness
Apr 6	Lamentations 3:55-57	Pit/ Quicksand
Apr 24	Ezekiel 34:11-16	Shepherd Sheep
July 1	Ezekiel 36:26-28	New Heart
Sept 1	Ezekiel 47:12	Leaves for Healing
Nov 25	Daniel 3:17	God Is Able
Feb 21	Daniel 6:22	Angel
Aug 5	Daniel 10:12,19	Do Not Be Afraid
Oct 24	Habakkuk 3:17-19	Yet I Will Exult Lord
Apr 18, Oct 31	Haggai 1:8	Rebuild Temple
Title Page	Malachi 3:16	Book of Remembrance
May 23	Malachi 4:2-3	Revere God's Name

June 5, Oct 31	Malachi 4:6	Father's Turn To Children
Aug 5	Several Passages	Do Not Be Afraid
Nov 25	Several Passages	God Is Able

NEW TESTAMENT

Feb 21	Matt 1:20	Angel
June 25	Matt 4:11	Angel
Oct 9	Matt 5:1-10	Be Attitudes
Mar 30	Matt 5:14-16	Light to World
Jan 6	Matt 6:9-13	Lord's Prayer
Jan 30	Matt 6:33,34	Seek First
Dec 1	Matt 7:7-8	Ask, Seek, Knock
Feb 2	Matt 7:24-27	House on Rock
Nov 25	Matt 9:28	God Is Able
Apr 5	Matt 10:1,5,7,8	Disciples Authority
Oct 31, Nov 17	Matt 11:28-30	Yoke Easy
Jan 30	Mark 12:28-31	Two Commandments
June 17	Matt 14:22-33	Boat
Apr 20	Matt 17:20	Move Mountains
Mar 13	Matt 25:34-40	Did to Me
Sept 21	Mark 4:36-41	Calm Storm
Nov 24	Mark 10:13-16	Jesus Touch Bless
Aug 8	Luke 1:30	Do Not Be Afraid
Aug 8	Luke 2:10	Do Not Be Afraid
Aug 8	Luke 5:10	Do Not Be Afraid
June 21	Luke 5:16	Kneeling
Sept 14	Luke 10:1-9, 17	Disciples sent
Sept 28	Luke 10:29-37	Good Samaritan
June 7	Luke 11:36	Smile Light
Apr 24	Luke 15:3,4	Lost Sheep
Dec 2	Luke 16:22	Angel
Aug 25	Luke 22:27,28	Learn to Serve
Oct 18, Nov 8	Luke 22:42-43	Angel
Sept 15	John 1:4,5	Light
Nov 6	John 2:6-10	Water Into Wine
Jan 3	John 4:14	Water
Jan 3	John 8:12	Light
Aug 17	John 8:31,32	Set Free
Aug 11	John 12:24	Wheat Dies
Oct 3	John 13:4-5, 12-17	Wash Feet
Sept 11	John 14:1-7	In Father's House
Mar 28	John 14:15-17	Holy Spirit Comforter
July 15	John 14:27	Peace I Leave
Grieving	John 14:27-29	Peace I Leave

May 6	John 15:15	Call You Friend
Apr 11	John 16:32-33	I Am Not Alone
Oct 2	John 21:3-6,11	Fishing
Mar 19	Acts 1:4,8	Wait
Aug 6	Acts 1:8	Power
Nov 9	Acts 3:1-8	Walking, Leaping
Nov 22,23	Acts 4:1-24	Peters Sermon
Nov 28	Acts 8:4-8	Healing by Philip
Dec 3	Acts 9:32-35	Healing by Peter
Dec 12	Acts 9:36-42	Dorcas Healed
June 25	Acts 12:7	Angel
July 20	Acts 19:11	Miracle
Aug 8	Acts 27:23-26	Do Not Be Afraid
May 2	Romans 5:3-5	Exult in Tribulations
Feb 24	Romans 8:25	Patience
Apr 26	Romans 8:18-25	Sufferings Hope
May 13	Romans 8:26-28	Spirit Prays
July 17	Romans 8:36-39	Nothing Separate
July 26	Romans 12:15	Rejoice/Weep
Oct 25	Romans 15:13	God of Hope
Apr 18	1 Corinthians 3:16	Temple God
July 24	1 Corinthians 9:24-27	Run Race
Sept 29	1 Corinthians 9:25	Crown
Dec 16,17	1 Corinthians 12:12-29	Body of Christ
Feb 12	1 Corinthians 13:4-7,13	Love
May 10	1 Corinthians 13:11	Child
Nov 14	2 Corinthians 1:3-11	Suffering = Comfort
July 3	2 Corinthians 4:7-10	Cracked Pot
May 29	2 Corinthians 4:11-18	Not Lose Heart
May 20	2 Corinthians 5:1-9	Groan in House
Nov 25	2 Corinthians 9:8	God Is Able
Apr 4	2 Corinthians 12:7-10	Thorn in Flesh
Dec 31	2 Corinthians 13:11-14	Finally, Brethren
July 5	Galatinas 5:22-23	Fruit of Spirit
Mar 3	Galatians 6:9	Spring Follows Winter
Sept 25	Galatians 6:9-10	Caregivers Prayer
May 27	Ephesians 3:14-19	Rooted in Love
Nov 25	Ephesians 3:20	God Is Able
Aug 3	Ephesians 4:31	Anger/Danger
May 10	Ephesians 6:11-18	Armor
July 18	Ephesians 6:16	Shield of Faith
Oct 23	Ephesians 6:10-20	Armor
Aug 9	Philippians 1:9-11	Filled
Jan 27	Philippians 2:1-4	My Joy Complete
Dec 19	Philippians 3:13-14	Run Race

Feb 10	Philippians 4:4-8,19	Rejoice Peace
Aug 6	Philippians 4:6,7	Peace
Aug 16	Philippians 4:11-13	Can Do All Things
Aug 6	Philippians 4:19	Provision
Aug 27	Colossians 1:3-5, 9-14	Not Cease to Pray
May 27	Colossians 2:6,7	Firmly Rooted
May 21	Colossians 3:2	Set Mind
Jan 10	Colossians 3:12-17	Put on
Jan 4	Colossians 3:16	Sing
Sept 29	1 Thessalonians 2:19	Crown
Aug 6	2 Timothy 1:9	Purpose
Nov 25	2 Timothy 1:12	God Is Able
Sept 29	2 Timothy 4:7,8	Crown
Jan 23	Titus 3:8	Speak Confidently
July 10	Hebrews 4:15,16	Throne of Grace
Dec 22	Hebrews 5:8	Learned Obedience
Nov 25	Hebrews 11:19	God Is Able
Nov 1	Hebrews 12:1	Cloud Witnesses
Aug 1	Hebrews 12:7-11	Discipline
June 23	Hebrews 12:12-13	Strengthen Knees
May 29	Hebrews 12:15	No Root Bitterness
June 8	James 1:2-8, 12	Testing Endurance
Sept 29	James 1:12	Crown
Jan 19	James 3:13-18	Wisdom
Mar 21	James 5:13-16	Call Elders
Mar 26	1 Peter 2:24	His Wounds
Aug 22, Oct 31	1 John 1:9	Forgive
May 26	1 John 4:4	Greater Is He
Aug 18	1 John 4:18	No Fear in Love
June 15	3 John 2	Good Health
Sept 1	Revelations 22:1-2	Leaves for Healing
Apr 28	Our Father	Count 10

MY WRITINGS

Jan 3/4	Discipline to Daily Devotional Life
Jan 8	Bread, New Man
Jan 12	Name
Jan 20	Butterflies are Free Fifty and free
Jan 26	Everlasting Arms
Feb 1	Holy Spirit Prayer
Feb 7	Saved
Feb 13	Love is Color of Rainbow
Feb 15/16	Wedding Vows/Hands on Bible, Job
Feb 20	Peanut Butter and Honey

Feb 22/23	Lost
Feb 25	Teammates Introduction
Mar 4	Silence
Mar 15	Light in Darkness
Mar 19	Wait
Mar 22	Women's Ecclesiastes
Mar 31	Confession
Apr 7	Road Construction
Apr 14	Waiting
Apr 17	It Is Well With My Soul
Apr 21/22	Easter Egg Hunt
Apr 29/30	Rain/Rainbow
May 7	Mother's Prayer
May 9/10	Which Body
May 15	New Garment
May 22	Lighten Burden/Golf Clubs
May 28	Weeds
May 30	Hand Bells
June 3	God's Viewpoint
June 10	Seven Days Messages
June 19	Father Prayer
June 27/28	Golf
June 30	Adoption
July 5	Choose/Fruits
July 12	Poison Water
July 19	Rocks
July 27/28	Shifting Gears
Aug 4	Bathroom Grout/I Know
Aug 6	Sweet P's Prayers
Aug 9	Refill Vessel
Aug 11	Let Go - Seeds
Aug 13	Add Faith to Life = Life
Aug 22	Sorry, Lord
Sept 8	Compassion
Sept 19/20	Half Time
Sept 22	Apple
Sept 24	Maze
Oct 31	Six R's
Nov 29	Names of God
Dec 6	Christmas House Cleaning
Dec 13	Silent Day
Dec 21	Fear Keeps Out Joy
Dec 24	Candle Light Service
Dec 26	Burned House
Dec 28	Christmas Cards

Post Script, Angel Experiences
Face to Face
Two Angels
Grieving
Final Word From the Lord

To Order ...

Send Check or Money Order To

Personal Word Ministries, Inc.
11309 E. 78th Terrace
Raytown MO 64138-2848

Set Free, A Caregivers Daily Devotional Journal	$18.00
Sales Tax	1.14
Shipping and Handling per book	3.00
Total	$22.14

Personal Word Ministries, Inc.

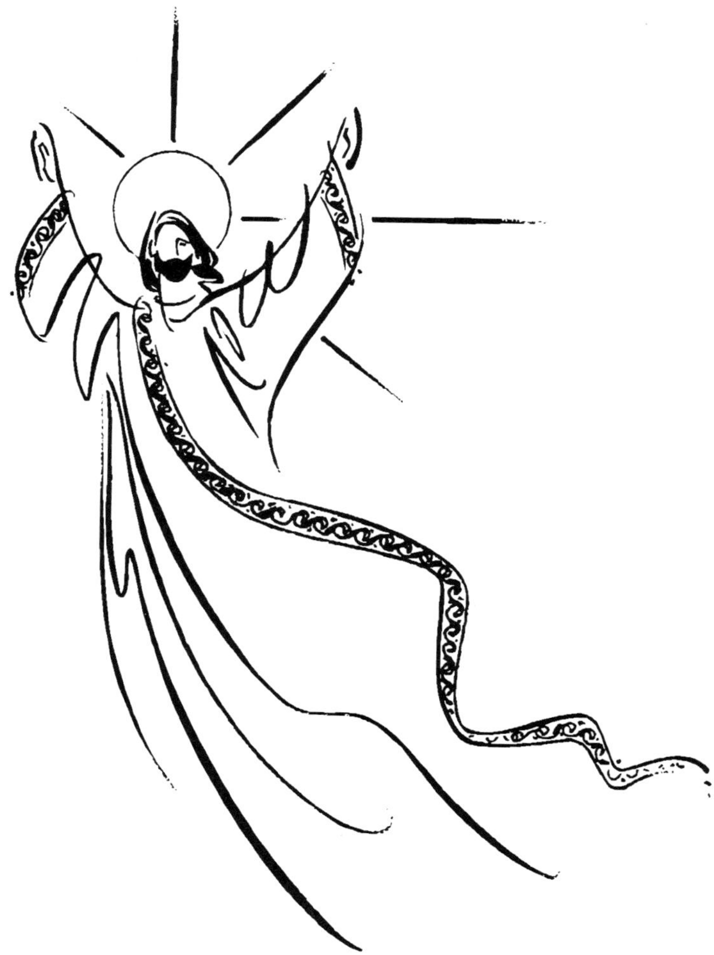

To Order ...

Send Check or Money Order To

Personal Word Ministries, Inc.
11309 E. 78th Terrace
Raytown MO 64138-2848

Set Free, A Caregivers Daily Devotional Journal	$18.00
Sales Tax	1.14
Shipping and Handling per book	3.00
Total	$22.14

Personal Word Ministries, Inc.

Final Word from the Lord. . .

From Chapters Three to Ten in the Book of Numbers

I, the LORD, have called Martha, a first-born, to be Mine.
I, the LORD, have called Martha's and Lily Publications' literary first born, *Set Free - A Caregivers Daily Devotional Journal* to be Mine.
I, the LORD, have called them to be set apart - wholly given to Me.

For seven years the *Journal* has been home schooled. This is now the **Suddenly Season** when the camp is to move out.

I, the LORD, have assigned and called by name those who are to do the work of serving and carrying the *Journal*.

I, the LORD, have called you who hold this *Journal* in your hands at this moment to move out towards the promised land of healing with these Words of Mine.

Move out as family and friends.
Move out as caregivers.
Move out as medical personnel.
Move out as support groups.
Move out as chaplains and pastors.
Move out as hospital gift shop and bookstore distributors.

On this twenty-second day of the second month of 1998 when the *Journal* was finished, I am anointing and consecrating it to be one of tools that will set the captives free from the slavery of illness and disease.

Two silver trumpets of Lily Publications and Personal Word Ministry are blowing and summoning the congregation to set out to go to war in the land against the adversary who attacks the body.

Move out singing the song of Moses,

> "Rise up, O LORD!
> And let Thine enemies be scattered,
> And let those who hate Thee flee before Thee."

Rest saying,

> "Return Thou, O LORD
> to the myriad thousands of Israel."

I am the LORD your God.

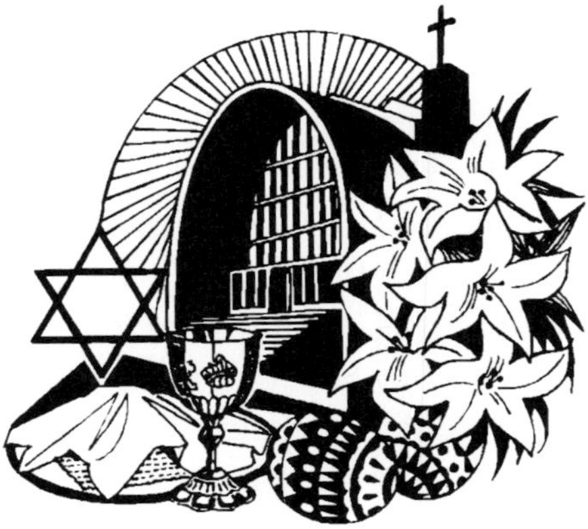

What Others Say . . .

Proverbs 25:11 says: "Like apples of gold in settings of silver is a word spoken in right circumstances."

Some of my most awkward moments have been when I have been in situations that I have not experienced. Martie has the ability to know the words to speak to those that are caregivers. This only comes from experience. Her *Caregivers Journal* is a compilation of words that minister to this group of people.

Steven H. Behrends, MD

Martie is an honest, transparent person who has learned in life that if she does not plant spiritual flowers in her garden, weeds will grow.

I encourage you to read, meditate, digest this work which was inspired by sorrow and the Holy Spirit to gain victory over "dis-ease" in life. You will prosper by this work of hope and victory.

Dr. Ray W. Hawk, Chiropractor

Thank you for sharing your *Caregivers Journal* with me. You must know how helpful it is to sit and share a few moments with the Lord when things get too heavy to bear. But you should also know that your *Journal* is helpful because it takes me on a fast spiritual journey when I'm tired and my head is fuzzy. Sometimes those are the best times to steal away.

I would think anyone seeking a respite could find something helpful in your words. It warms my spirit to know that someone else has "been there, done that" when I am feeling lonely and bogged down by the little things.

Ann O'Donnell, Caregive